IMAGES
of America

The MEDEX Northwest Physician Assistant Program

On the Cover: John Betz and Paul Snyder, graduates of MEDEX Class 1, trained and worked in Othello, Washington, with their preceptors—Drs. Richard Bunch and Kenneth Pershall. The two physician assistants (PAs) served Othello as providers and preceptors for over 40 years. Snyder retired in 2012 and Betz in 2014. From left to right are Betz, an unidentified female colleague, Snyder, and Dr. Pershall. (Courtesy of the MEDEX collection.)

IMAGES
of America

The MEDEX Northwest Physician Assistant Program

Ruth Ballweg MPA, PA-C

ARCADIA
PUBLISHING

ISBN 978-1-4671-3480-4

Published by Arcadia Publishing
Charleston, South Carolina

Printed in the United States of America

Library of Congress Control Number: 2015942517

For all general information, please contact Arcadia Publishing:
Telephone 843-853-2070
Fax 843-853-0044
E-mail sales@arcadiapublishing.com
For customer service and orders:
Toll-Free 1-888-313-2665

Visit us on the Internet at www.arcadiapublishing.com

This book is dedicated to Richard Smith, MD, MPH, in recognition of his role in creating MEDEX Northwest as a model for health workforce development.

Contents

Acknowledgments

This book would not have been possible without the support, patience, and attention to detail of Mary Giles, MEDEX archivist. The author also acknowledges the assistance and support of the Society for the Preservation of Physician Assistant History, the specific MEDEX faculty and staff members who have supported and encouraged this process, and the individual PAs and PA programs that responded to requests for photographs and information. Special thanks go to faculty, staff, and graduates of the MEDEX program who have historically continued to demonstrate Dr. Smith's principles for increasing access to health care through a collaborative model of education, advocacy, and inclusion.

Unless otherwise noted, all images used in this book come from the MEDEX collection.

The following individuals and organizations generously donated additional images: the Richard Smith collection; the DENTEX collection; the MEDEX Alaska collection; the Physician Assistant History Society Archive of Johns Creek, Georgia; Willie Foster, of Group Health Cooperative Archives; University of North Dakota Physician Assistant Program; Rauner Special Collections, Dartmouth University; Dr. Donald Pedersen, University of Utah Physician Assistant Program; Shelly Powers, Howard University; Charles R. Drew Physician Assistant Program; Fred Hutchinson Communications; University of Washington Office of Graduate Medical Education, Dean of Medicine; Clare McLean/UW Medicine; MEDEX faculty and staff; and Larry Applebee, Laurie Benton, Chris Carson, Machelle Dotson, Gary Goldfogel, Leslie Howard, Ian Jones, Nanette Laufik, Scott Light, the Lurie family, Joe Marzucco, Susan "Reba" McIntyre, Robin Moore, Jane Perry of the University of Worcester, Dawanda Pesicka, Chad Tiller, Kurt Welser, and John Winklmann.

INTRODUCTION

As we prepare to celebrate the 50th anniversary of the physician assistant profession in 2017, this book tells the story of the University of Washington's MEDEX Northwest Physician Assistant Program, which, as the nation's second physician assistant program, adapted the new health profession to serve the unique health-care needs of the Pacific Northwest beginning in 1967.

The history and success of the University of Washington's MEDEX Northwest Physician Assistant Program is all about remarkable people: the altruistic and innovative physicians who sought to improve health care in the Pacific Northwest, the young returning military corpsmen willing to take a chance on an unproven career path, and the supportive patients who valued the care that these young men provided. Generous physicians provided lectures and welcomed MEDEX students into their practices. Courageous leaders in the School of Medicine and the Washington State Medical Association introduced legislation that allowed PAs to practice and incorporated young PA leaders into their infrastructure. Hardworking MEDEX faculty and staff members adapted the curriculum over time and promoted the PA career domestically and internationally. For over 45 years, MEDEX graduates—now men and women from many prior health careers—have pioneered new roles for physician assistants and made a difference in the lives of their patients. This book is their story.

Created by Dr. Richard Smith in 1967, MEDEX Northwest was designed to not only build a new health career for individuals with prior health-care experience, but also to be a catalyst for social justice in American medicine. The first students were returning military corpsmen from the war in Vietnam. Regardless of what Americans felt about the contentious war, they had seen the impact of these well-trained corpsmen in caring for the troops. When the corpsmen came home, there was national interest in guaranteeing that their medical skills would not be lost. Emerging PA programs such as the Duke Physician Assistant Program in 1965, followed by MEDEX in 1967, showed the country how military medical skills could be applied in a variety of civilian settings.

A graduate of Howard University Medical School, Dr. Smith initially joined the US Public Health Service as a member of the Epidemic Intelligence Service, and later served in Nigeria as a medical director for the fledgling Peace Corps. Pres. Lyndon Johnson then assigned Dr. Smith to lead the federal initiative to desegregate the US hospital system as a requirement for Medicare reimbursement. After his successful leadership of this difficult task, Dr. Smith asked Surgeon General Dr. William Stewart to assign him to the University of Washington. His goal was to establish MEDEX based on what he had learned from health-worker models in Cuba and Africa.

Working collaboratively with the Washington State Medical Association, MEDEX immediately focused on solving a serious health-care access problem: the departure of isolated and overworked physicians from practices in rural Washington. In addition, MEDEX was also a chance to demonstrate new models of care in large urban health systems. Seattle's Group Health Cooperative trained and employed four members of MEDEX Class 1 as a strategy to expand care in its rapidly growing system. With an emphasis on diversity in its recruitment and selection process, MEDEX was able to place and retain culturally competent graduates in order to accommodate a wide range of clinics providing care to medically underserved patients.

The infrastructure of MEDEX/physician assistant practice required—and still requires—a legal relationship with a specific supervising physician as a condition for practice. With prior experience as military corpsmen, new MEDEX graduates were immediately able to assume significant responsibilities in primary care, emergency, and surgical settings. Extensive research and evaluation methodologies were built into MEDEX in order to demonstrate a wide acceptance by physicians and patients.

As PA programs developed across America, one of the main issues became what to call the graduates. At Duke, they were called physician associates; in Washington, they were called Medex, and in Colorado, they were child health associates. The American Medical Association weighed in as well with strong opposition to the term "associate." They felt the term was too collegial and did not give a strong enough message that the physician was in charge.

There were some major differences—and points of tension—between the various training models. Duke centered its training in hospitals, MEDEX focused on primary care, and the Colorado program directed its energies toward the care of children. A program at the University of Alabama at Birmingham provided training specifically in surgery. In addition, the four-year Alderson Broaddus program in West Virginia offered a bachelor's degree to its young students with no prior health experience. The three-year program in Colorado provided a master's degree to students who often had already worked with children.

Representatives of the founding institutions soon began communicating about their educational models. Included were Duke University, the University of Washington, the University of Colorado, Alderson Broaddus College, and the University of Alabama at Birmingham. The American Academy of Physician Assistants (AAPA) was established in 1968. Program directors established the Association of Physician Assistant Programs (APAP), now the Physician Assistant Education Association (PAEA), in 1972. In 1973, AAPA and APAP sponsored a landmark conference in Wichita Falls, Texas, that brought the various models of the profession together under the common umbrella of the AAPA.

Simultaneously, national organizations and processes were developed to deal with the issue of program accreditation and the certification of individual PAs. The National Commission on Certification of Physician Assistants (NCCPA) was established in Atlanta in 1972. The Joint Review Committee for Educational Programs for the Assistant to Primary Care Physicians (JRC-PA) grew out of other accreditation programs housed in the American Medical Association's Chicago headquarters in 1971. New PA graduates from Duke (William Stanhope), MEDEX (Steven Turnipseed), and Colorado (Loretta Ford) represented the interests of PAs in the creation of both the Accreditation Review Committee on Education for the Physician Assistant (ARC-PA) and the NCCPA. ARC-PA became a freestanding organization in 2000 and is now also headquartered in Atlanta.

Eventually, all of the programs agreed that the new profession should be unified with the name "physician assistant." There were several iterations of this over time to include "physician's assistant," indicating possession. Even now, some PAs still believe that the title should be changed to "physician associate," which is probably a better description of the role, and was chosen by PAs in the United Kingdom and New Zealand in 2014. In the United States, however, the physician assistant title is so embedded in federal and state laws and administrative rules that it would be extremely difficult to change. The AAPA's current view is that physician assistants should be called simply by the initials "PA," much as "RN" is used to designate registered nurses.

State PA academies were created as programs developed. The Washington Academy of Physician Assistants (WAPA) has remained closely tied to the Washington State Medical Association (WSMA) and is housed in the WSMA offices, where it also contracts for legislative and policy support by the WSMA lobbyists. Many MEDEX faculty members and graduates have served as presidents and officers over the years.

Within the University of Washington health-sciences programs, a spin-off of public-health programs resulted in the creation of the new School of Public Health in 1970 soon after MEDEX began. With the leadership of Dr. Robert Day, the School of Public Health dean, MEDEX moved into the School of Public Health along with other programs such as health services, epidemiology, biostatistics, and environmental health. Dr. David Lawrence became the second MEDEX program director and worked to further develop the program and integrate MEDEX with other health profession programs at the University of Washington. (Dr. Lawrence later became the national chief executive officer of the Kaiser Permanente system.)

The physician program directors who followed Dr. Lawrence were pediatrician Dr. Carole Jenny, who is now a national expert on child abuse; Dr. Robert Harmon, who later served as the administrator for the Health Resources and Services Administration and a leader within United Healthcare; and Dr. Andrew Penman, the chief executive officer of the Cancer Council of New South Wales.

Despite the support of organized medicine, the future for PAs remained uncertain into the 1980s. In 1982, the federal government issued a landmark policy document by the Graduate Medical Education Advisory Committee. The committee reported that there would be an excess of 70,000 doctors in the United States by 1990 and recommended that medical schools decrease their class sizes by 10 percent. While few medical schools followed their guidance, there was a major impact on federal funding for physician assistant and nurse practitioner (NP) programs. MEDEX, which had relied almost exclusively on federal funding, had to find other funding sources or close its doors.

While MEDEX needed a stable funding source, three other programs within the University of Washington, including two within the School of Public Health, faced a similar crisis. The School of Public Health, the School of Business, and the School of Engineering banded together to create the first University of Washington "self-sustaining programs." After the approval of the Board of Regents and the Washington state legislature in 1981, this new status allowed four programs, which included MEDEX, to determine their own class sizes, set their own tuition rates, and retain most of their tuition income for program operations. While MEDEX still successfully competed for federal funding, it was economically stable for the first time in its history. Later, during the 1990s health reform period, the Washington state legislature provided specific funding to expand PA educational opportunities in Eastern Washington.

From 1986 to the present, MEDEX has received $8.9 million in federal funding from Health Resources and Services Administration agencies, including PA Training Grants, the Health Career Opportunities Program, the Office of Rural Health Policy, and Model Education Projects for the Health Professions.

With stable funding, the program rapidly developed by extending the length of training and adding clinical training opportunities in addition to its traditional one-on-one family medicine preceptorship. While MEDEX students had been eligible for a bachelor's of general studies degree from the University of Washington, a new MEDEX-specific bachelor's of clinical health services (BCHS) degree was created in 1986. The first BCHS degree was awarded to John Yerxa, who later served as a MEDEX clinical coordinator and faculty member. MEDEX remained in the School of Public Health until 1994, when it was transferred back into the School of Medicine—first in the Department of Medical Education and then, in 2011, the Department of Family Medicine.

In the 1980s and 1990s, the PA profession finally stabilized as PAs began to take over the leadership of PA programs, and clinically experienced PAs took major responsibility for all aspects of PA education. Physician presence was ensured by the ARC-PA requirement that all programs have a medical director who reported to the program director. Ruth Ballweg (Class 11) was the first PA to be appointed MEDEX program director in 1985. When MEDEX joined the Department of Family Medicine in 2011, Terry Scott (Class 25) was appointed program director and Ruth Ballweg was moved up to a new role as section chief. Terry Scott was named section chief and program director in July 2015.

A major federal breakthrough occurred when the 1997 Balanced Budget Act finally assured Medicare reimbursement for both physician assistants and nurse practitioners. This major recognition brought credibility and permanence that had previously been lacking.

Back in the School of Medicine, MEDEX expanded geographically within the Washington, Wyoming, Alaska, Montana, and Idaho (WWAMI) medical education region to include decentralized training sites in Sitka, Alaska (1993), Yakima, Washington (1994), Spokane, Washington (1997), Anchorage, Alaska (2009), and Tacoma, Washington (2013).

In response to the ARC-PA requirement for all PA programs to offer master's degrees by 2021, MEDEX worked with the University of Washington's graduate school to develop two master's degrees, one in clinical health services and the other an extended master's degree in clinical health services for practicing physician assistants. By 2015, MEDEX offered master's degrees in Seattle and Spokane and bachelor's degrees in Anchorage and Tacoma. By 2021, all sites will offer master's degrees.

MEDEX has expanded its visibility and its influence to include ad hoc membership in the Executive Committee of the School of Medicine, its Clinical Chairs Group, and participation in the WWAMI Regional Affairs Group. By 2015, over 200 PAs were employed within the University of Washington medical system.

Nationally, the PA profession has attained high visibility. *Forbes* named the physician assistant degree the number-one master's degree for employment in 2015. *Forbes* had previously ranked PAs in the top five jobs for more than 10 years. *Forbes* based its decision on the projections of the Bureau of Labor Statistics and the increasing need for PAs during the era of health reform, as well as the overall flexibility of the career. Other business and medical management publications have provided similar coverage to the growing PA profession. By 2014, the National Commission on Certification of Physician Assistants reported that it had certified the 100,000th PA.

MEDEX students stand out from many other programs because of the continuing requirement for prior clinical practice. MEDEX also continues to enroll an equal number of men and women due to active recruitment of military and community-based men and women. The average age of MEDEX students has consistently been 32–35. The recruitment strategy also involves encouraging clinics and hospital systems to identify qualified employees and facilitate their application for eventual rehire. While MEDEX's generalist curriculum emphasizes primary-care employment, MEDEX graduates are also employed in every medical specialty.

The PA profession is being adapted to meet the health-care access needs of multiple countries, and MEDEX is involved in many of these developments. The Netherlands has been the most successful and efficient in implementing both physician assistants and nurse practitioners. By 2015, there were 900 PAs practicing throughout the Netherlands with full licensure and prescriptive practice. For Commonwealth Countries, the standard practice was to develop a "pilot" before moving ahead with full recognition of the profession. The United Kingdom, Scotland, the province of Ontario in Canada, the Australian states of Queensland and South Australia, and New Zealand all completed pilots using PAs from the United States and have gone on to have varying degrees of acceptance of the career. MEDEX graduates have served in all of the pilots with the exception of Ontario. African countries such as Ghana and South Africa directly established programs to serve their specific needs. In the process, MEDEX has become involved in many of these developments and has hosted visitors from Australia, New Zealand, British Columbia, Ontario, China, Ghana, South Africa, Mozambique, the United Kingdom, and Scotland.

Ultimately, the real story of MEDEX is about the many people who have worked together to change the face of health care in the Pacific Northwest. In August 2015, the program had 2,233 graduates—most of whom serve in the WWAMI region. This book tells their tale.

One

The Collaborative Model of MEDEX Northwest

As the physician assistant profession emerged between 1965 and 1970, each of the founding PA programs had a specific niche to fill. For MEDEX, the priority was addressing the burnout of rural physicians in America's Northwest. These isolated doctors were working too hard without backup and had little time for continuing medical education or for their families. Another niche explored was the effective integration of the MEDEX model into large health-care systems, such as Health Maintenance Organizations (HMOs) and Group Health Cooperative, that emerged on the West Coast during the 1950s

MEDEX founder Dr. Richard Smith was key to the program's design and success. At his own request, he was sent to Washington by Surgeon General Dr. William Stewart. Dr. Smith wanted to prove that his use of trained clinical support personnel while in the Peace Corps in Africa could be applied to improve health-care access in the United States. He strategically gained the support of both the University of Washington School of Medicine and the Washington State Medical Association (WSMA) as cosponsors of MEDEX.

Dr. Smith actively recruited military corpsmen returning from Vietnam as the first students. He also employed two innovative physicians, Dr. Raymond Vath and Dr. Gerald Bassett, as the program's co-leaders and identified a former military corpsman, William Freeman, as the role model for the new career. As part of his strategic plan, he asked members of the WSMA to serve as future mentors of program graduates, to participate on the admissions committee, and to sponsor legislation that allowed PAs to practice in Washington.

Over time, the MEDEX team developed an innovative and efficient curriculum to train primary-care providers. They spent time preparing rural communities in Eastern Washington to receive and fully use these new providers, convinced rural physicians' wives that their husbands would be home for dinner if they hired Medex graduates, and trained the students how to best fit into their new communities.

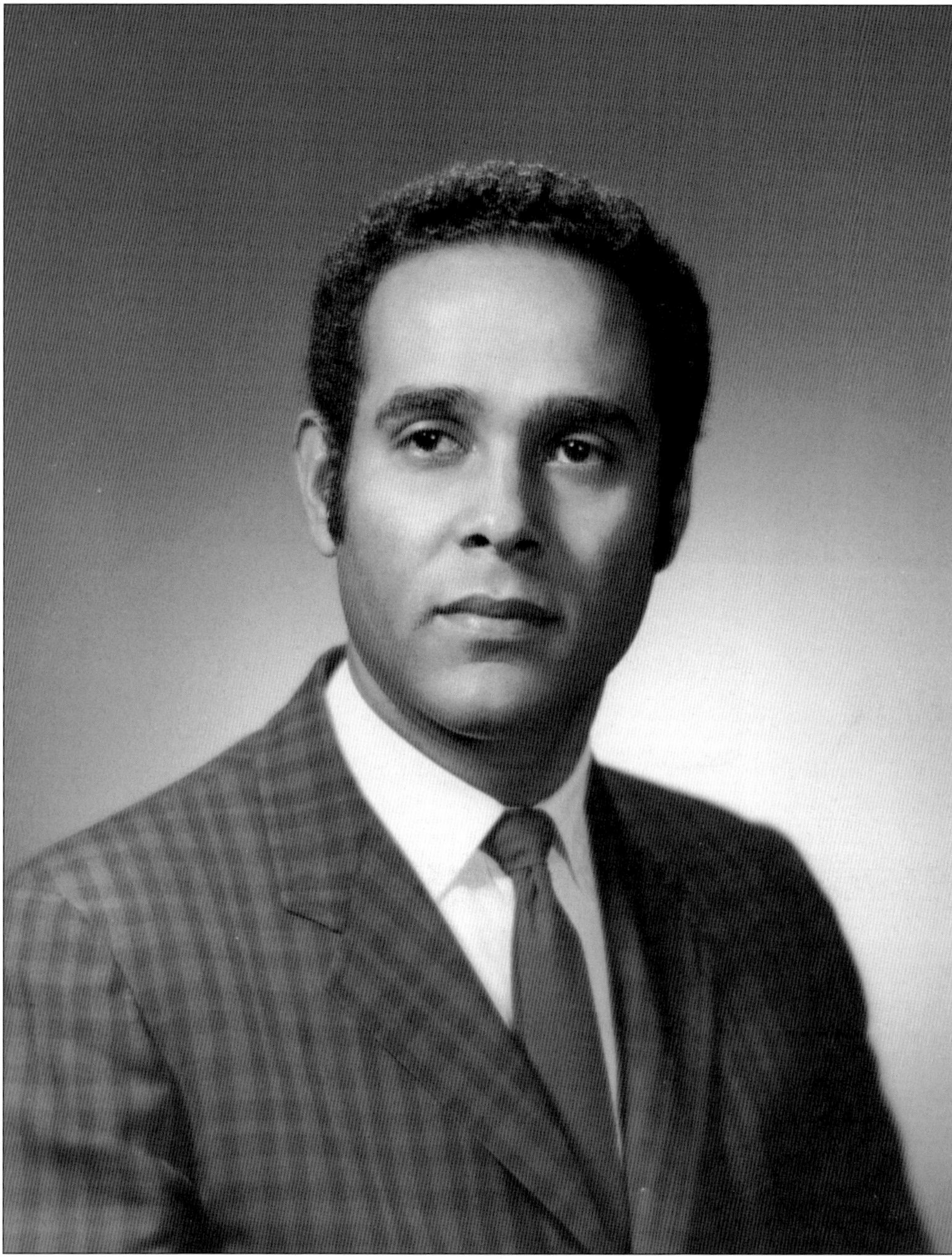

MEDEX FOUNDER. A Howard University School of Medicine graduate, Dr. Smith was also trained in public health. As a US Public Health Service officer, Dr. Smith served in the Epidemiology Intelligence Service, then as Peace Corps medical officer for Africa. He was called back from Nigeria to lead a federal initiative to desegregate US hospitals as a requirement for Medicare reimbursement. He was then relocated to Seattle to develop MEDEX. (Courtesy of the Richard Smith collection.)

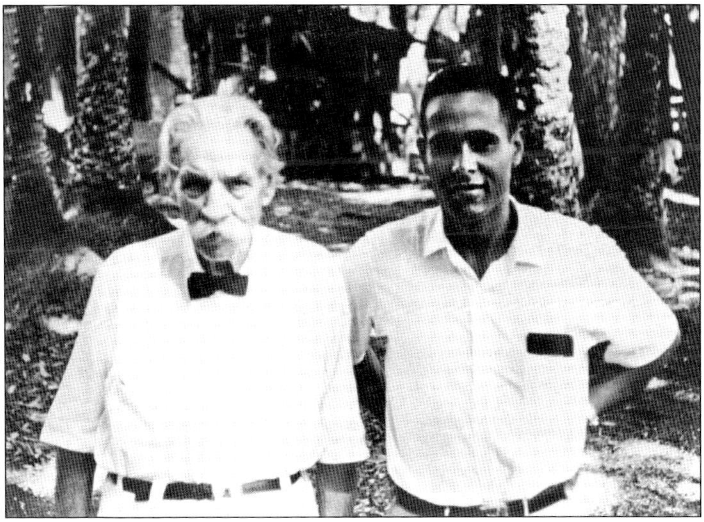

Drs. Schweitzer and Smith. While in Africa, Dr. Smith met with Dr. Albert Schweitzer (left) to discuss their common love of music and also to get feedback about his idea of improving health-care access using a new category of health provider. Dr. Schweitzer was not encouraging. (Courtesy of the Richard Smith collection.)

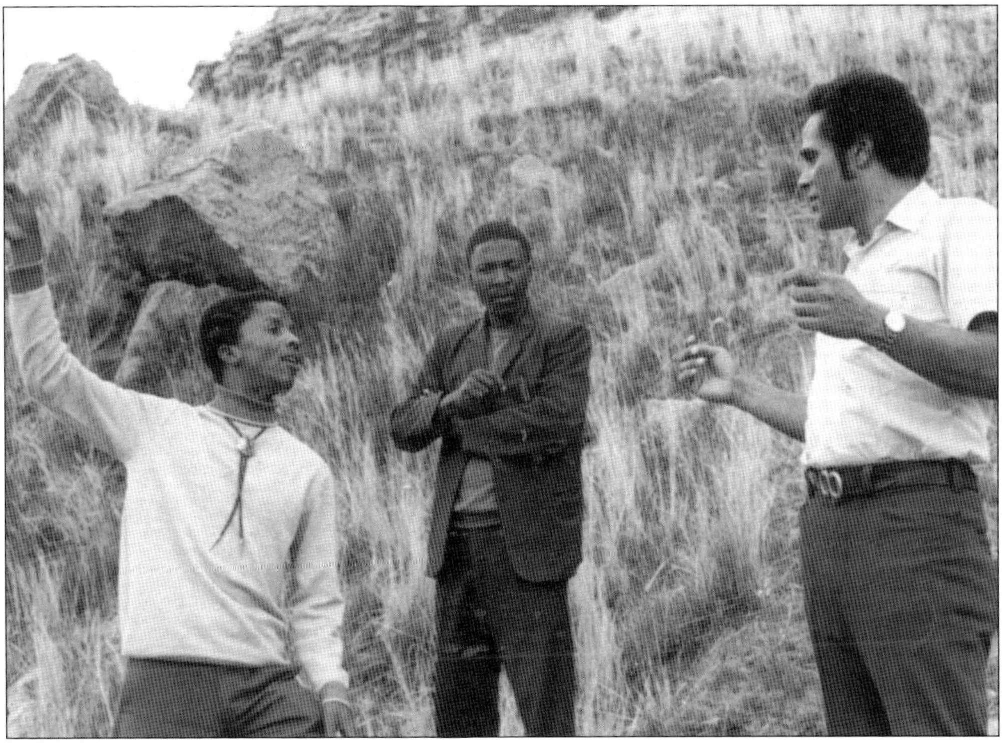

Dr. Smith and African Health Workers. Dr. Richard Smith and two African health workers are seen discussing clinical problems in their region. Dr. Smith created his MEDEX model based on non-physician clinical roles he had seen in Cuba and Africa. After completing his Peace Corps and hospital desegregation assignments for the US Public Health Service, he requested assignment to Seattle to promote and implement his idea for MEDEX. (Courtesy of the Richard Smith collection.)

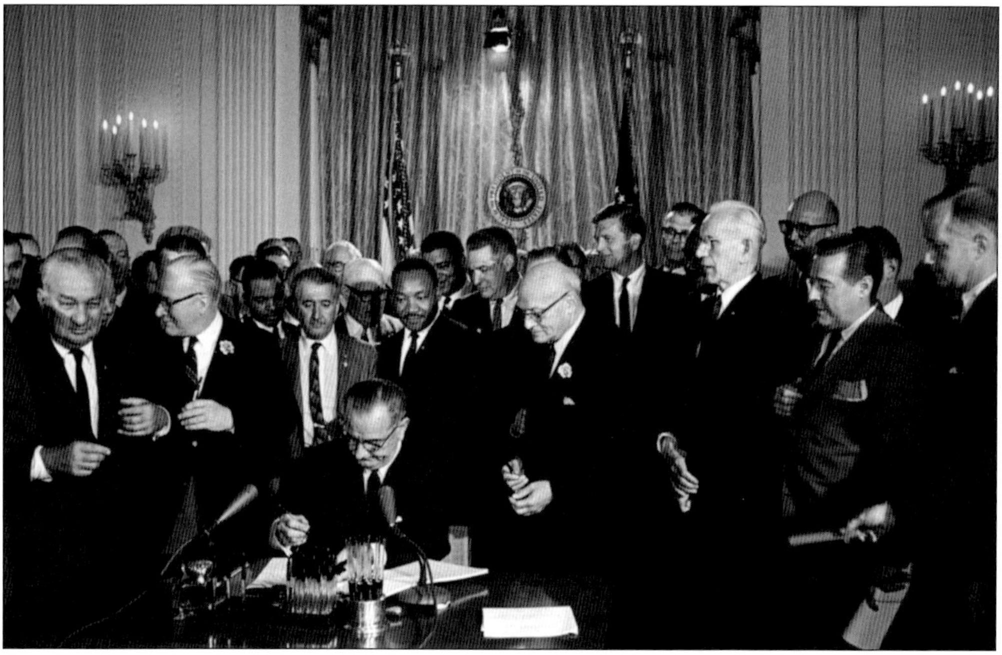

Civil Rights Act. The 1964 Civil Rights Act facilitated health-care access to disenfranchised Americans. Dr. Smith believed that access would involve the introduction of new health-care roles. Here, Pres. Lyndon B. Johnson signs the Civil Rights Act as Dr. Martin Luther King Jr. and others look on. (Courtesy of the LBJ Presidential Library.)

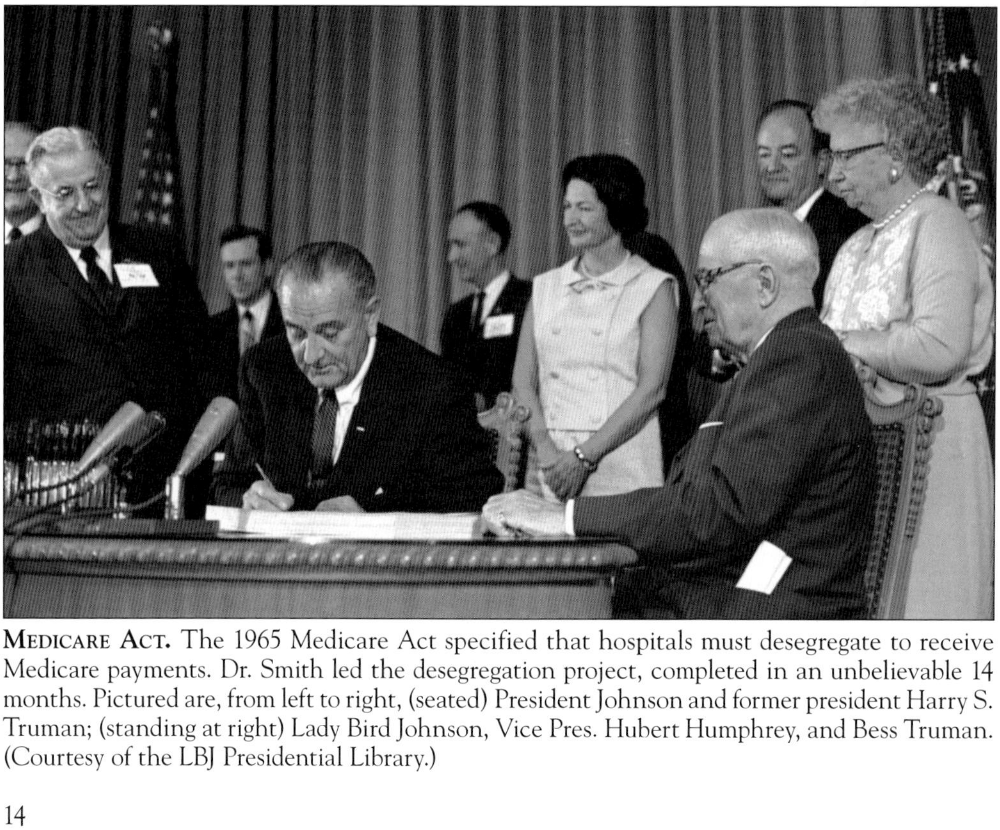

Medicare Act. The 1965 Medicare Act specified that hospitals must desegregate to receive Medicare payments. Dr. Smith led the desegregation project, completed in an unbelievable 14 months. Pictured are, from left to right, (seated) President Johnson and former president Harry S. Truman; (standing at right) Lady Bird Johnson, Vice Pres. Hubert Humphrey, and Bess Truman. (Courtesy of the LBJ Presidential Library.)

Dr. Smith's Communication Style. Dr. Smith (right) engages Dr. Ray Vath in conversation. Dr. Smith was a persuasive communicator with many media contacts. His visible passion and enthusiasm for his work convinced policy makers and motivated his coworkers. One of his consistent messages was that MEDEX graduates would "multiply the hands" of doctors in the practices and health systems that employed them, thus dramatically increasing access to health care.

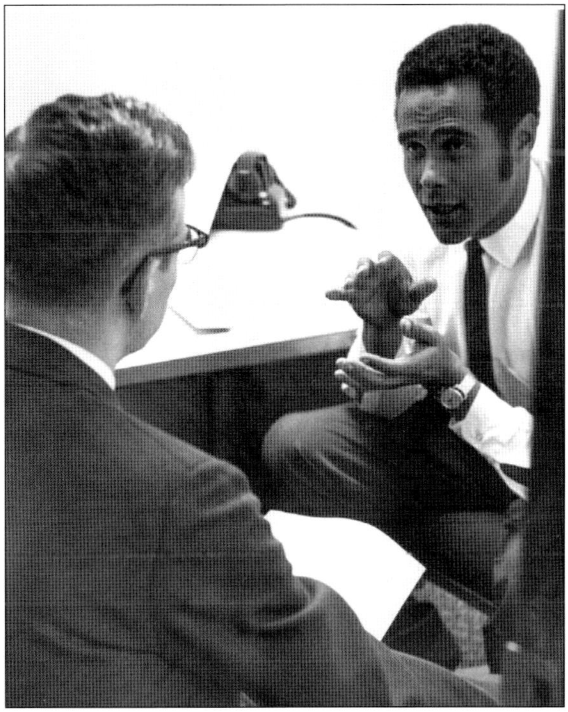

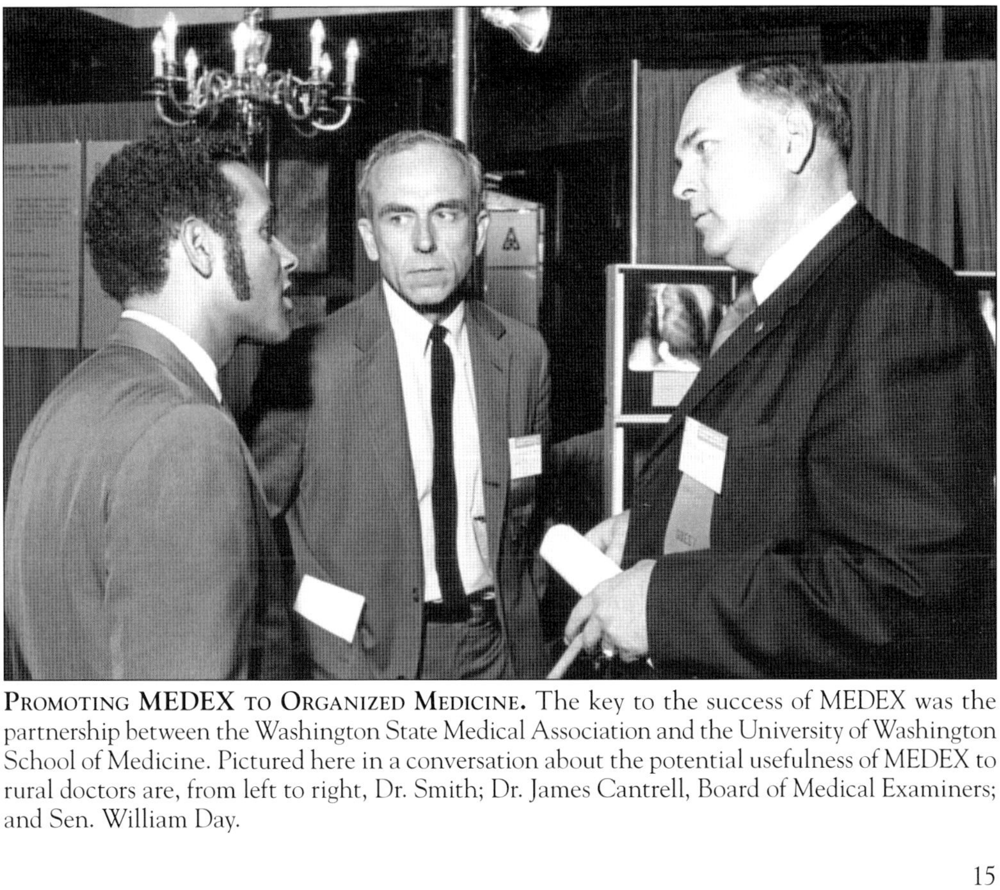

Promoting MEDEX to Organized Medicine. The key to the success of MEDEX was the partnership between the Washington State Medical Association and the University of Washington School of Medicine. Pictured here in a conversation about the potential usefulness of MEDEX to rural doctors are, from left to right, Dr. Smith; Dr. James Cantrell, Board of Medical Examiners; and Sen. William Day.

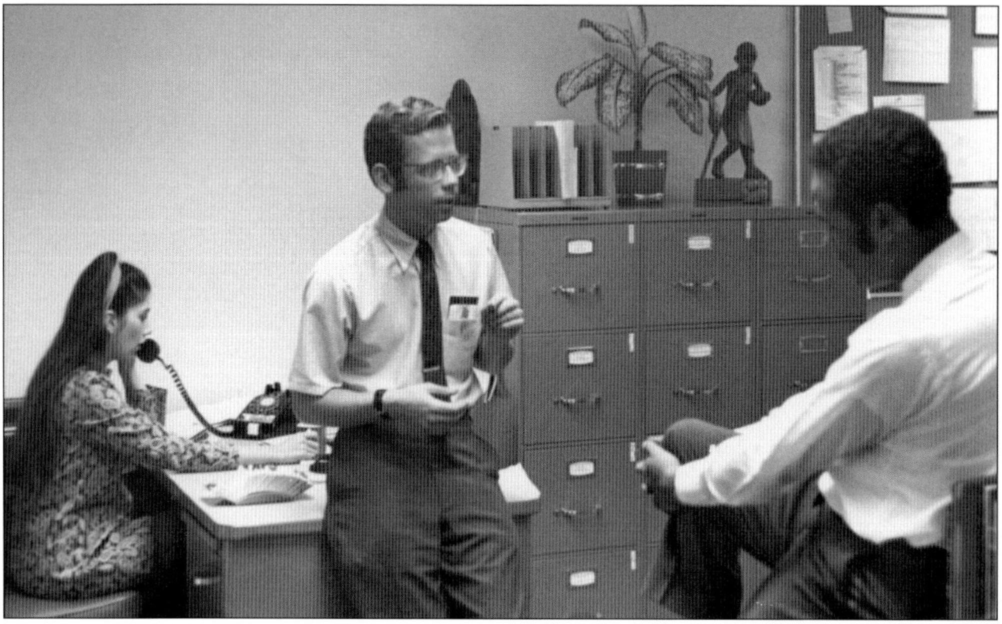

MEDEX Staff Support. Dr. Smith believed that assembling a strong staff was the key to the success of any project. Here, Dr. Smith is speaking with Lorna Carrier and Bill Freeman. Freeman—a former military corpsman himself—provided valuable input into the curriculum design. Later, Freeman went to medical school and served in the Indian Health Service in numerous clinical, leadership, and advocacy roles.

MEDEX—A Name and a Title. In choosing a name for the profession, Dr. Smith believed that using consonant-stop sounds, particularly *k* or *x*, would impart a strong, decisive image. To coin the term "Medex," he combined the French words for "physician extender." "Medex" in lowercase was both the title and form of address for the new practitioners; "MEDEX" in uppercase was the name of a specific training program.

Dr. Smith's "Systems" Concept. The intensive 18-month MEDEX training included didactic lectures and clinical experience with a primary-care preceptor. It united trainees, sponsoring doctors, clinical practice staff, and the surrounding community in a unique collaboration, with orientation, training, and outreach support for all involved.

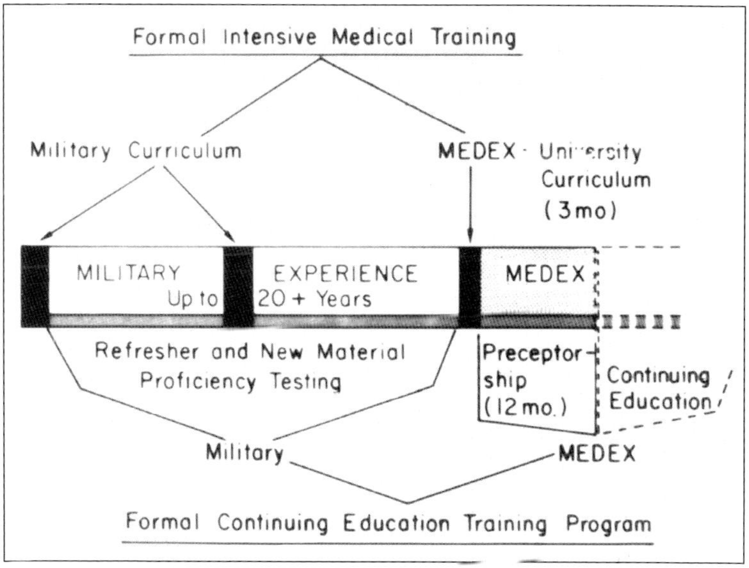

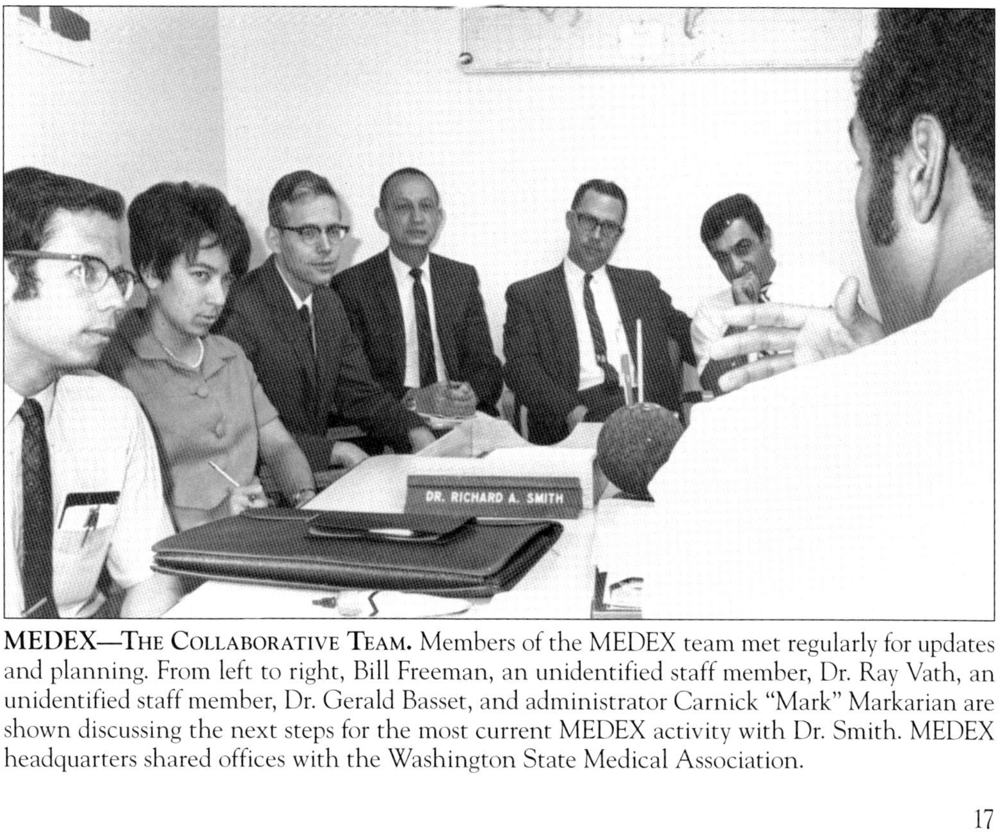

MEDEX—The Collaborative Team. Members of the MEDEX team met regularly for updates and planning. From left to right, Bill Freeman, an unidentified staff member, Dr. Ray Vath, an unidentified staff member, Dr. Gerald Basset, and administrator Carnick "Mark" Markarian are shown discussing the next steps for the most current MEDEX activity with Dr. Smith. MEDEX headquarters shared offices with the Washington State Medical Association.

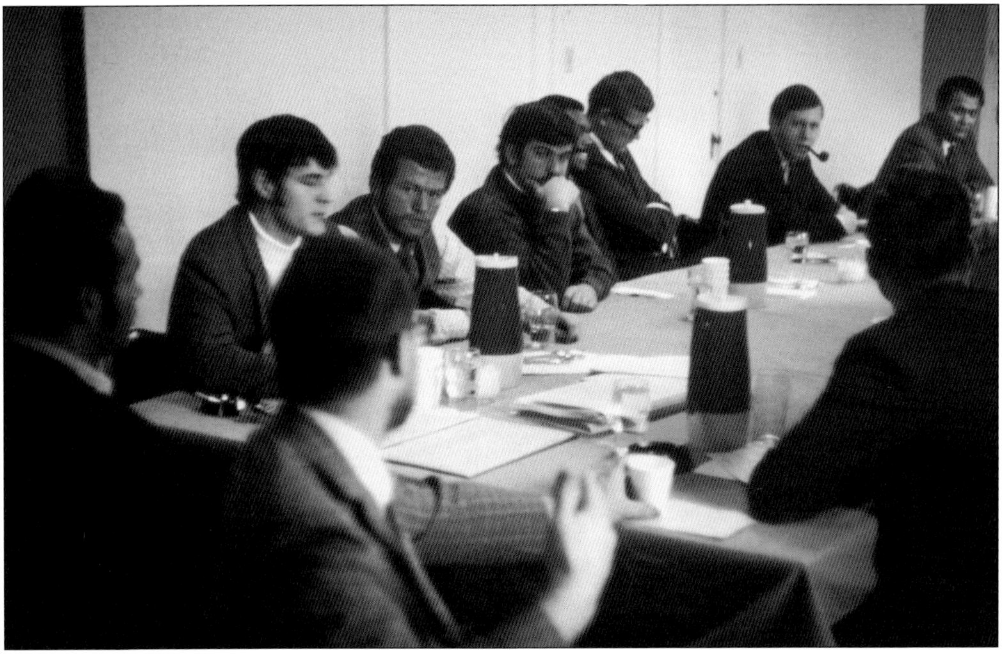

MEDEX Admissions Interviews—The Candidates. The MEDEX team designed a unique admissions process based on Dr. Smith's experience in the Peace Corps. Candidates, including those shown here, had group interviews and the opportunity to interact with the MEDEX staff and their future supervising physicians. The interview process also included activities for spouses.

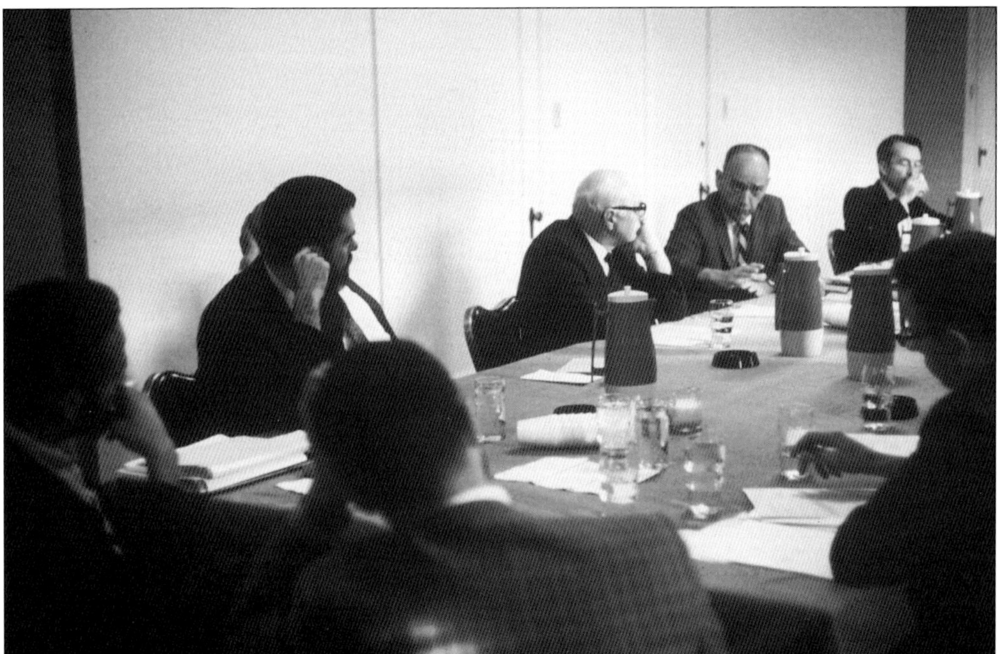

MEDEX Admissions Interviews—The Preceptors. In the early days of the program, precepting doctors had a crucial voice in assessing candidates.

MEDEX AT GROUP HEALTH. Dr. Robert Monroe of Group Health Cooperative in Seattle served as the preceptor for William Coleman (Class 3) and other MEDEX graduates. Group Health was the only urban site used by MEDEX initially, and provided an opportunity for the PA role to be trained in an early HMO.

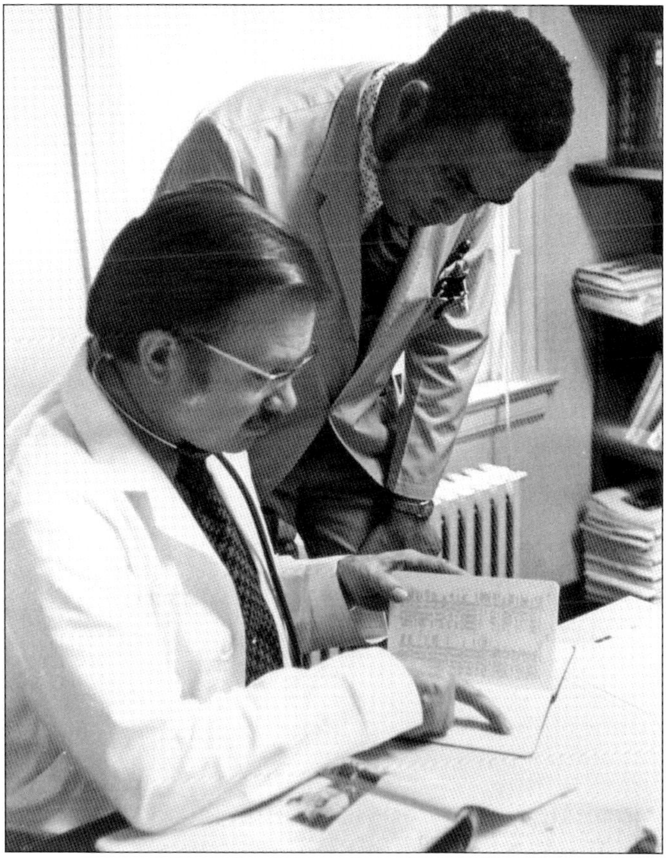

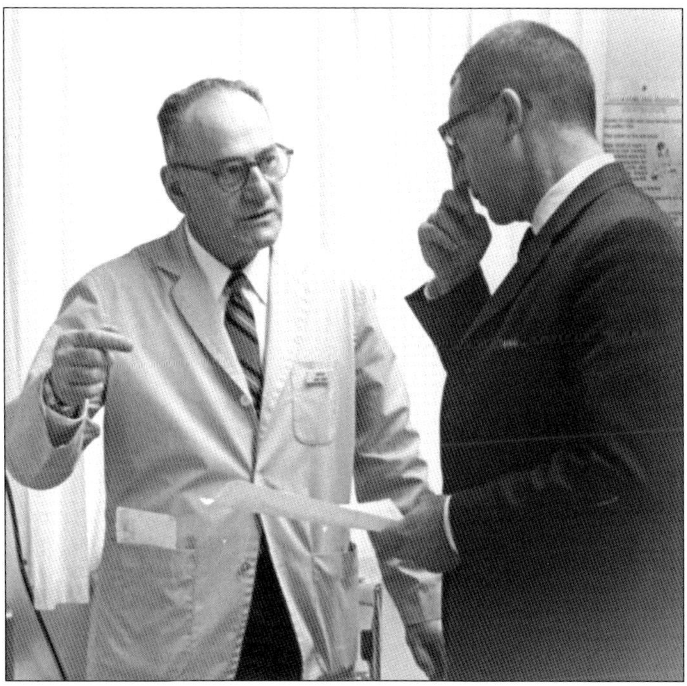

COLLEAGUES IN COLLABORATION. Students depended on close teamwork with the program, preceptors, and other students. Louis LeBert (Class 1), in distinctive Medex blue coat (left), confers with Loren "Carl" Chillquist (Class 1). As a medic, LeBert supervised medical training at Fairchild Air Force Base in Washington. Chillquist began in a Minnesota one-room schoolhouse and saw great possibilities in the Army Medical Corps. Later, he encouraged VA officials to hire his civilian-trained classmates.

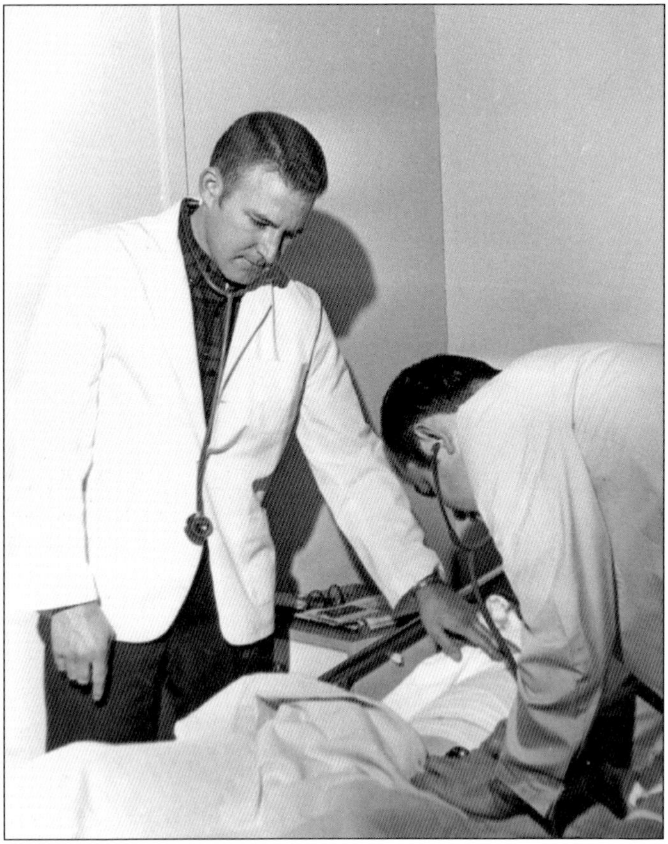

MEDEX in Northeast Washington. Dr. Marshall Thompson (left) and MEDEX student Ronald Graves (Class 1) collaborate in Davenport, Washington. The community gave a warm welcome to Graves; photos of the two men as a team were used in MEDEX media releases.

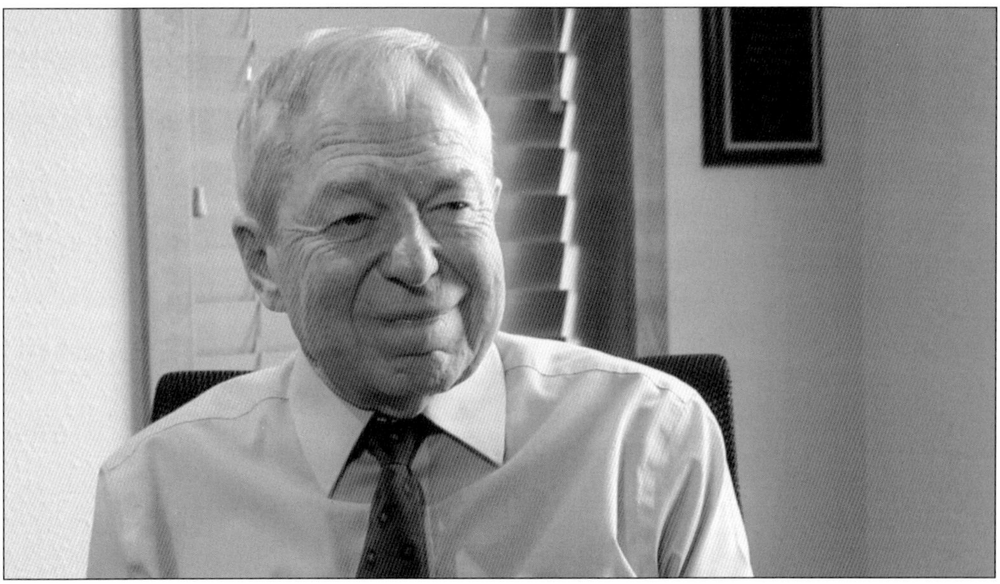

MEDEX in Central Washington. Dr. Richard Bunch, a physician in Othello, Washington, recruited both Paul Snyder and John Betz to his rural community by taking them hunting and fishing. As he said, "I figured you two guys already knew medicine, so I wanted to know if you'd fit!" Dr. Bunch is shown here in 2014.

Two

Early MEDEX Graduates

The success of MEDEX depended on the first class. They had to be flexible. They had to be smart. They had to be willing to be in the public eye. They had to be able to get along with everyone, including those who did not support them. They had to be willing to be the role models for all who followed in their paths. It was a tough job. Fortunately, Dr. Richard Smith's principles for creating a new career included some important lessons he had learned in the Peace Corps.

The first step was a highly visible recruitment process. Advertising in the military newspaper *Stars and Stripes*, Dr. Smith and his team created lots of interest among potential applicants. Over 500 military corpsmen applied. "New technology"—a room-sized computer donated by Seattle's Boeing aircraft company—helped to store and sort the applications. Washington State Medical Association board members and future physician-supervisors for the new MEDEX chose the first class. The unique interviewing process, modeled after Peace Corps processes, included a full day of interviews with rotating groups of candidates interviewed by groups of physicians. The interview day included a social session and interviews with the applicants' wives. The process was both memorable and stressful. Fourteen candidates were chosen to be Washington State's first physician assistants. The results were highly publicized, and there were many people, both pro and con, who wondered what would happen next!

Based on Dr. Smith's plan for a highly visible start-up, the MEDEX students were followed closely by the media both locally and nationally. With new PA programs at Duke University and the University of Washington, national magazines such as *Reader's Digest*, *Time*, and *Look* featured articles on the new career. The public was strongly supportive, having seen military corpsmen functioning in some highly stressful settings in American's "first televised war."

Placed in rural communities and in Seattle's Group Health Cooperative, members of the first MEDEX class were well received by doctors and their patients.

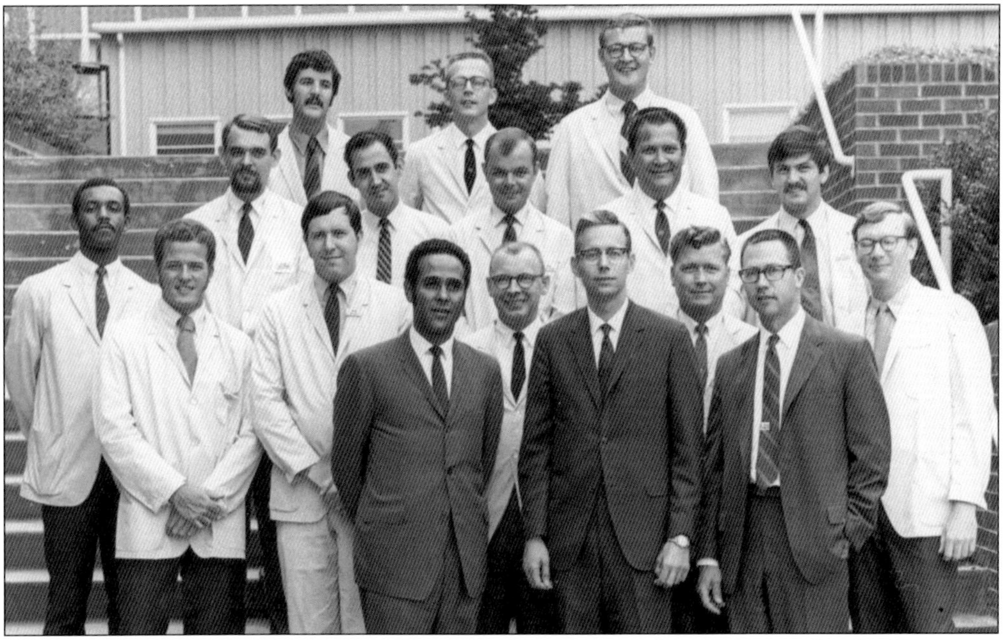

MEDEX Class 1: the Cohort. Members of the first MEDEX class are pictured at the University of Washington Health Sciences Center in their 1969 official class picture. In addition to the students, the photograph includes (from left to right in dark jackets) Dr. Richard Smith, Dr. Raymond Vath, and Dr. Gerald Basset.

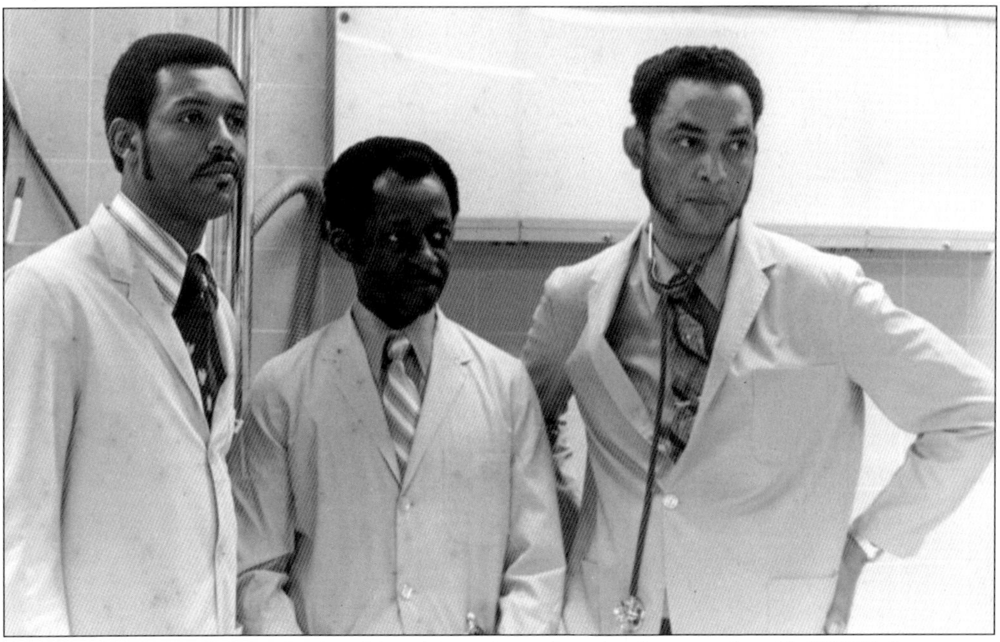

Diversity in MEDEX. Dr. Richard Smith's goal was that the demography of MEDEX classes—in contrast to that of medical schools—would match the diversity of America's population. Fortunately, the population of military corpsmen was very diverse, which helped in meeting this goal. Shown here are, from left to right, Steve Turnipseed (Class 1), Charles Phillips (Class 2), and William Coleman Jr. (Class 3).

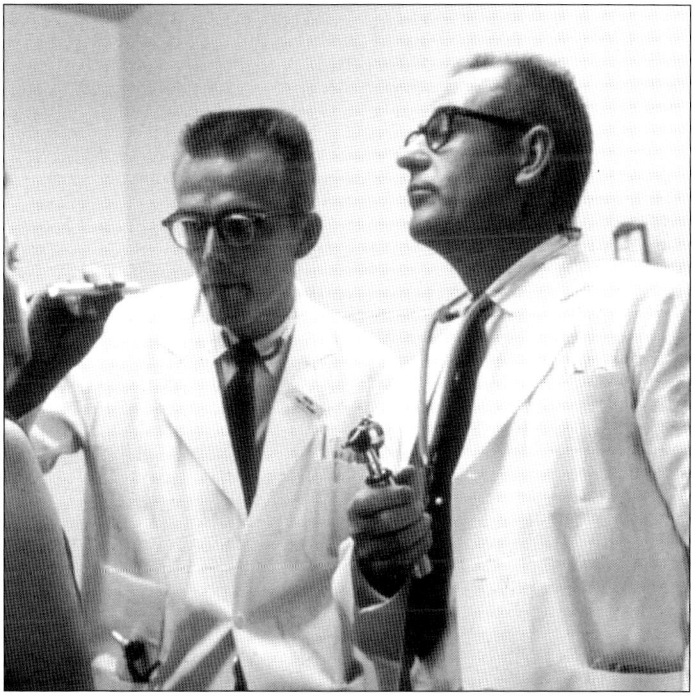

The Physician/Medex Partnership. The generalist educational model for MEDEX included a year of full-time one-on-one practice with a primary-care physician. In the late 1960s and early 1970s, family doctors, especially those in small towns, provided a broad range of care including general surgery, obstetrics, orthopedics, and emergency medicine. MEDEX Class 1 student Paul Snyder is pictured in Othello, Washington, with his supervisor and teacher Dr. Kenneth Pershall.

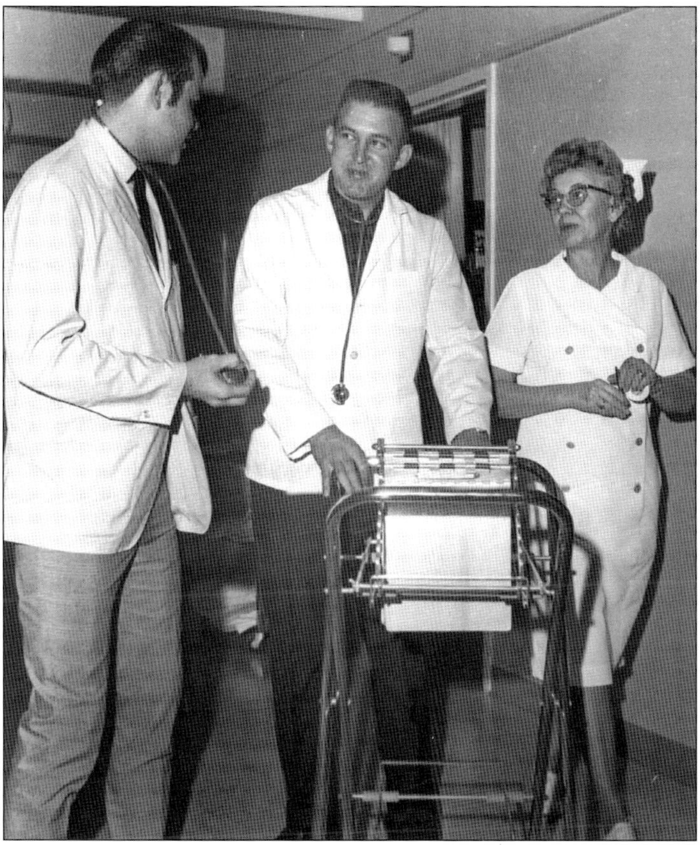

The Patient-Care Team. The MEDEX model included training of the entire clinical team to work together in support of the new role. Here, Medex student Ron Graves (left) is pictured during morning hospital rounds with his preceptor Dr. Marshall Thompson and an unidentified director of nursing.

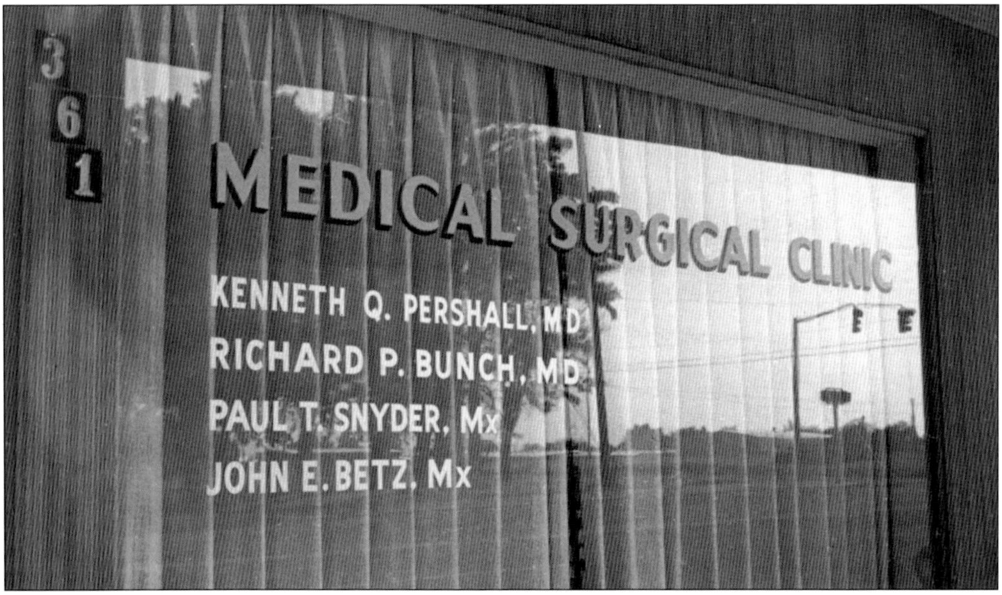

Recognizing Medex Practice. The introduction of the new clinicians into the community required that they be clearly identified and recognized within the practice. This included public welcoming activities in rural communities, clearly identified signage, and appropriate nametags and introductions with each patient at the beginning of each patient's visit. The Othello, Washington, practice of Dr. Richard Bunch and Dr. Kenneth Pershall clearly identified Medex John Betz and Medex Paul Snyder as members of the team.

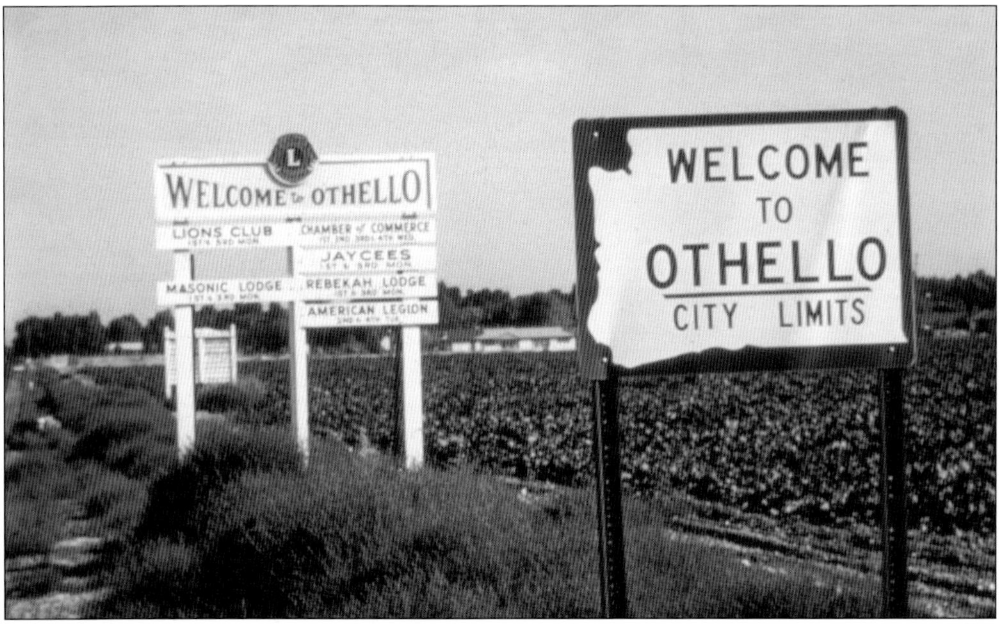

Rural Washington. Othello is a small community in Central Washington, described as the "heart" of the federal Columbia Basin dam and irrigation project. Agriculture is the major employer. Dr. Richard Bunch and Dr. Kenneth Pershall chose two members of Class 1, John Betz and Paul Snyder. The grads were quickly integrated into all aspects of community life, and the team received extensive media coverage, including a CBS special in 1970.

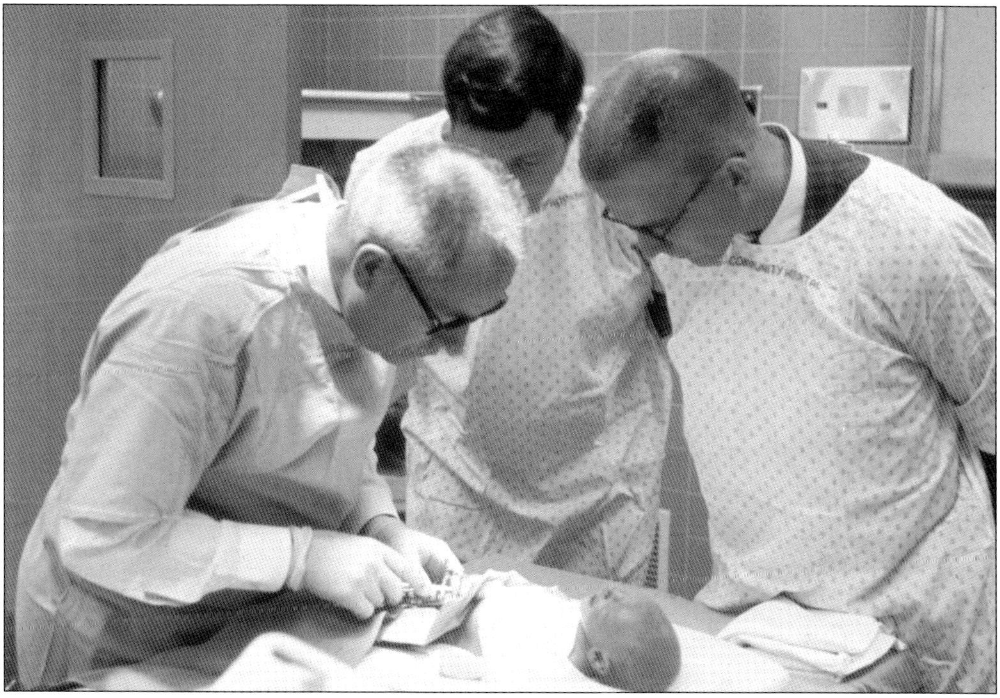

The Training Continues. In Othello, family medicine included a busy obstetrics service. From left to right, Dr. Kenneth Pershall, Medex John Betz, and Medex Paul Snyder (both Class 1) examine a medical model to review principles of infant care.

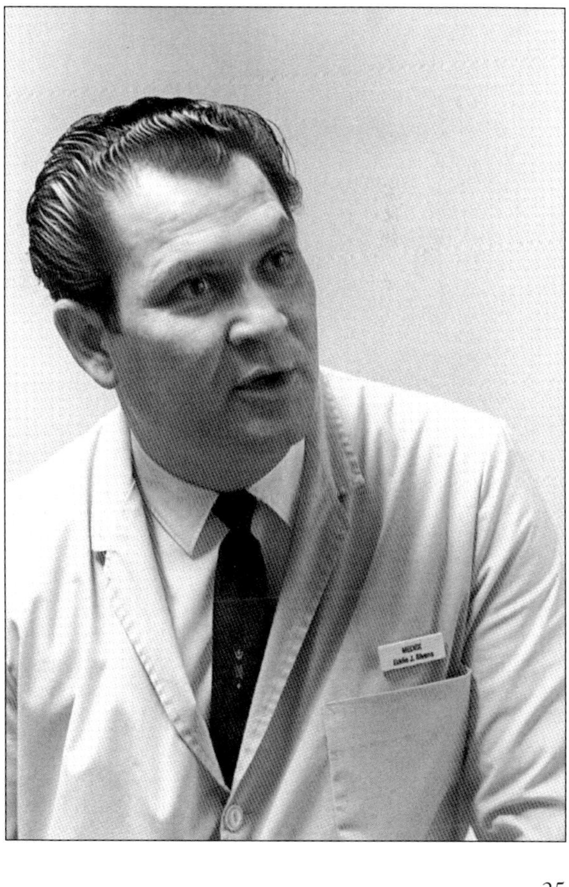

On the Columbia River. Medex Eddie Bivens (Class 1) worked with Dr. Wayne Henkle in White Salmon, Washington. With his military service background treating casualties in Vietnam, Bivens began right away to provide valuable assistance with surgical aspects of Dr. Henkle's practice.

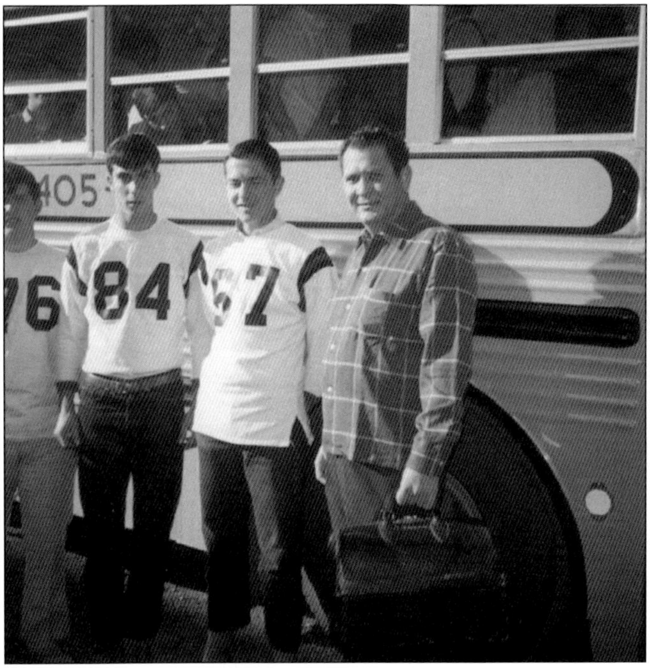

Expanded Roles and Community Involvement. Eddie Bivens is shown boarding a bus with members of the White Salmon football team. In addition to his busy clinical practice, Medex Bivens also provided medical coverage for the community's athletic teams.

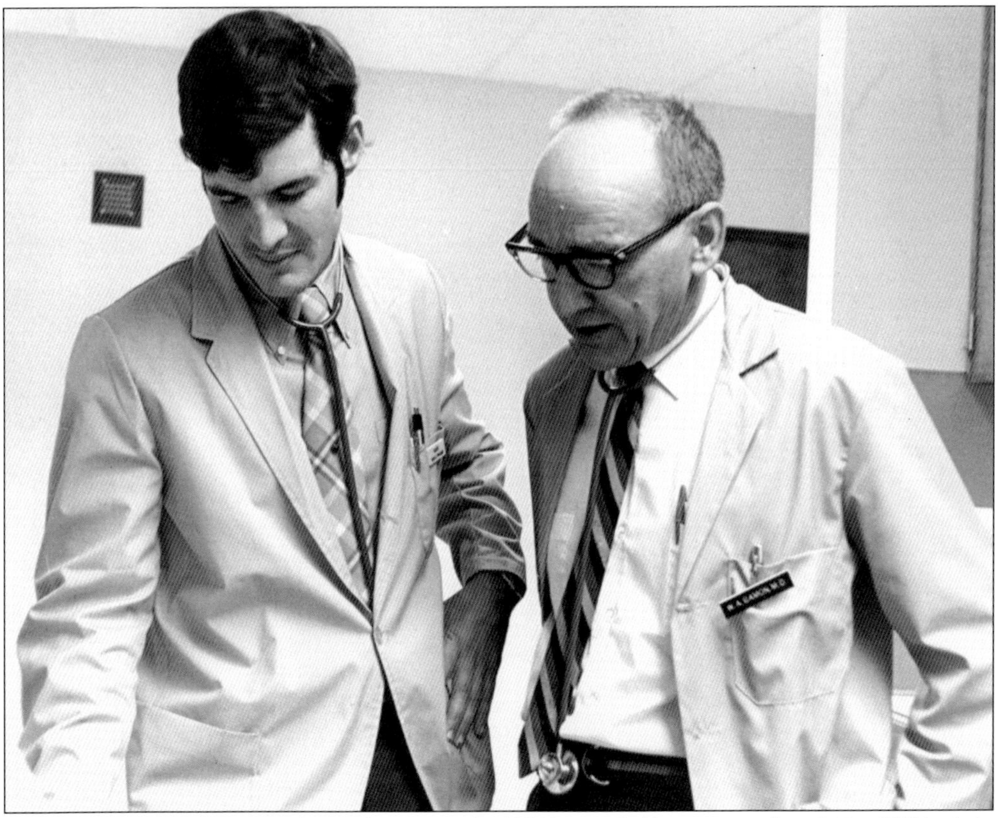

Eastern Washington. Medex Robert Woodruff (Class 1, left) is pictured with Dr. Wilfred A. Gamon in Cheney, Washington, a small college community.

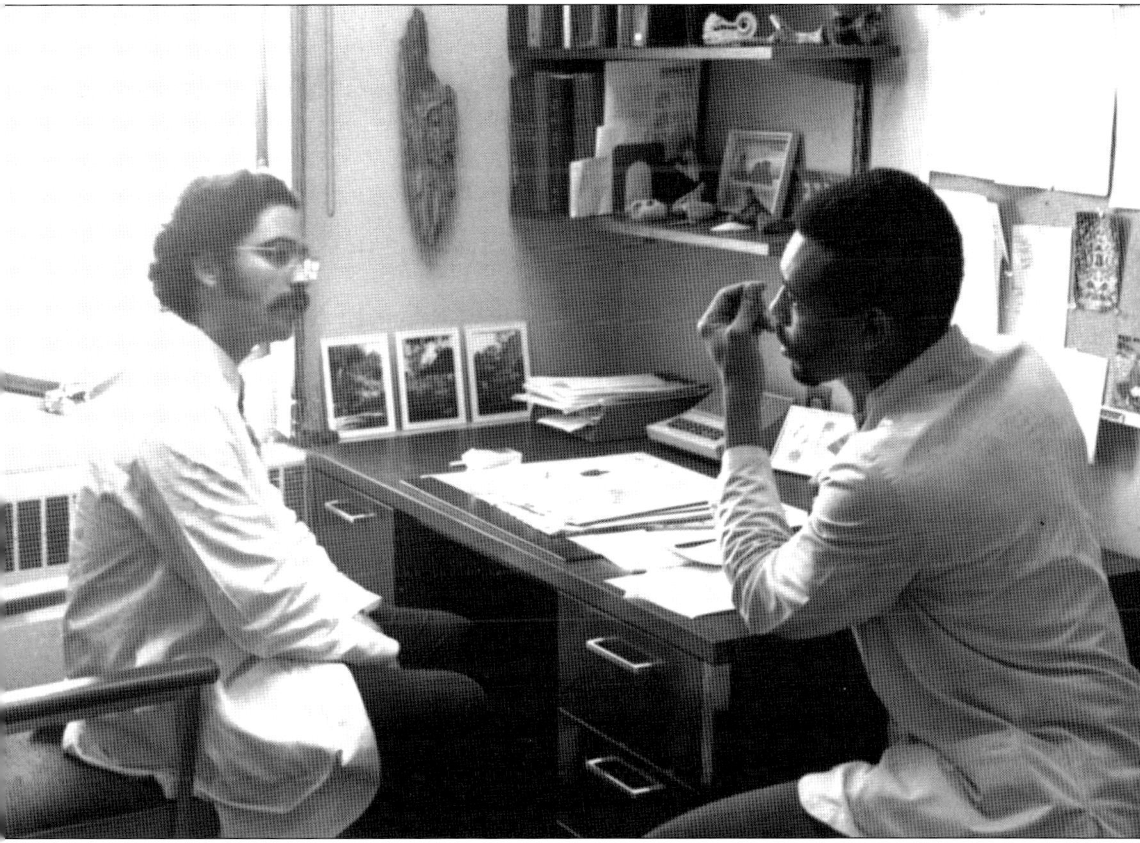

MEDEX AT GROUP HEALTH. Seattle Group Health Cooperative and its record of innovation made it an ideal partner for MEDEX and military corpsmen. The first Group Health PAs included Steven Turnipseed, Michael Carraher, and Thomas Coles (all Class 1), and William Coleman (Class 4). The new practitioners found enthusiastic acceptance. At the time, Group Health policy was that after three office visits with a Medex, patients were offered an appointment with their primary-care doctor. But patients typically chose to continue seeing the PAs, expressing confidence that "their Medex" would consult doctors as needed. Here, Turnipseed is shown consulting with social worker Ronald Croda (later Class 11). Turnipseed advanced to a leadership role at Group Health and served as president of the Washington Academy of Physician Assistants. (Courtesy of Group Health Cooperative Archives.)

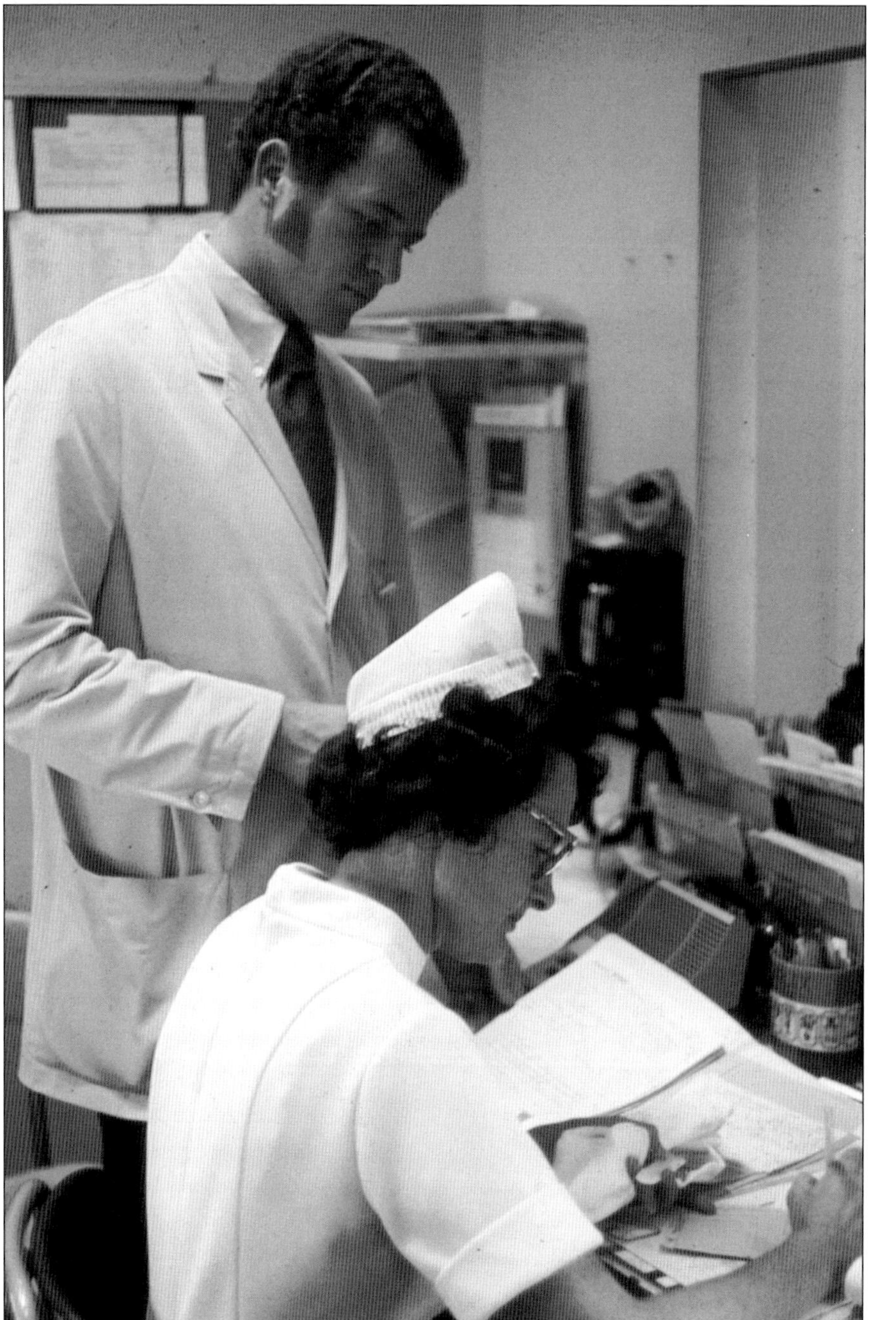

Coles at Group Health. Group Health incorporated Medex graduates throughout the organization. Trainees were especially useful—and visible—in the emergency room; their battlefield experience enabled fast, efficient care for a range of injuries. Thomas Coles (Class 1) is shown here with an ER nurse. Later, Coles went on to join Dr. Richard Smith as a trainer for MEDEX International, developing curriculum and training support for health workers in many countries around the world. In 1985, he received a Distinguished Service Award from the University of Washington's School of Public Health.

SUPERVISION AND OVERSIGHT. Medex Frank Ball (Class 4, left) is shown at Group Health with his preceptor Dr. Robert Bond. The photograph illustrates the close contact for mentoring, oversight, and advice that was provided by the supervising doctors who employed the early Medex. The MD/Medex team received formal instruction about how best to support each other. At the same time, the new clinicians were also given significant autonomy in working with patients.

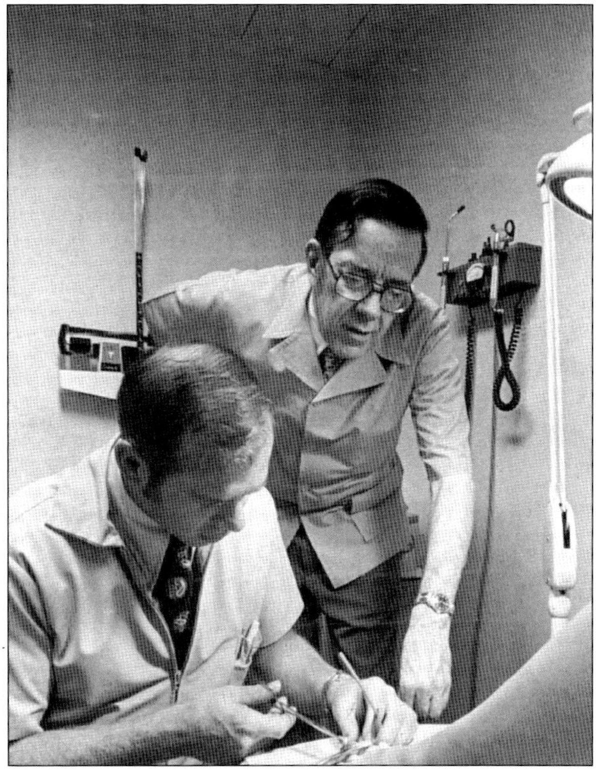

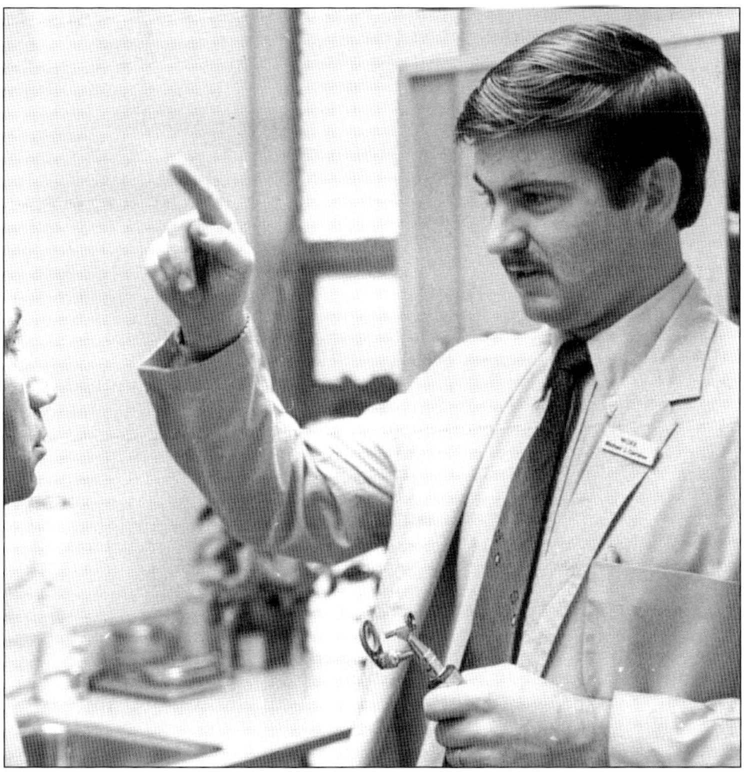

MICHAEL CARRAHER AT GROUP HEALTH. MEDEX students received extensive preparation in physical diagnosis. This instruction built upon the strong foundation of their prior military medical training. Here, Medex Michael Carraher is shown performing a thorough eye examination as part of a comprehensive physical in the office of preceptor Dr. Robert Sherry at Group Health Capitol Hill.

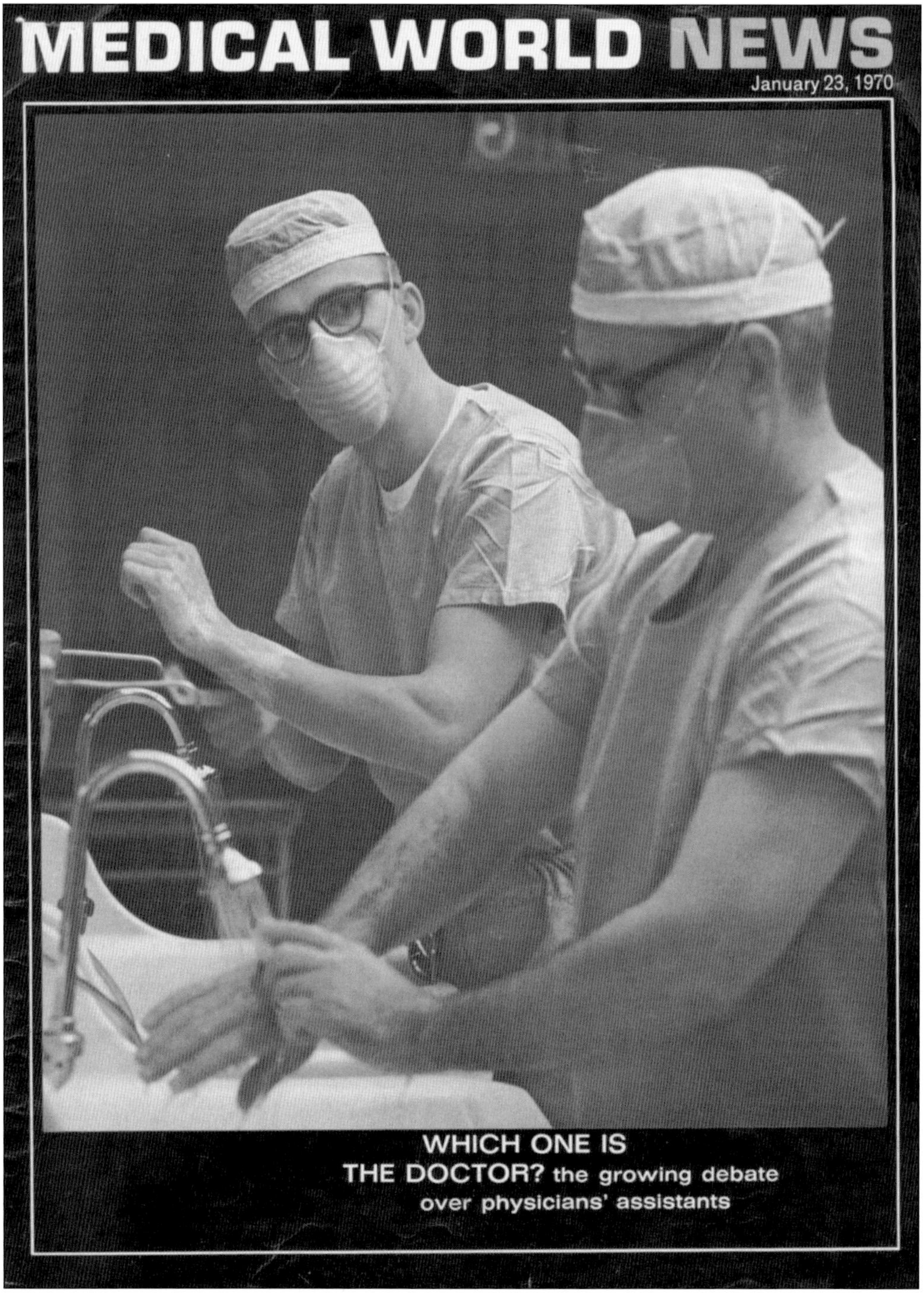

"WHICH ONE IS THE DOCTOR?" PA role development made headlines in publications such as this 1970 issue of *Medical World News*. Here, Class 1 graduate Paul Snyder (left) scrubs in for surgery with preceptor Ken Pershall, MD (right).

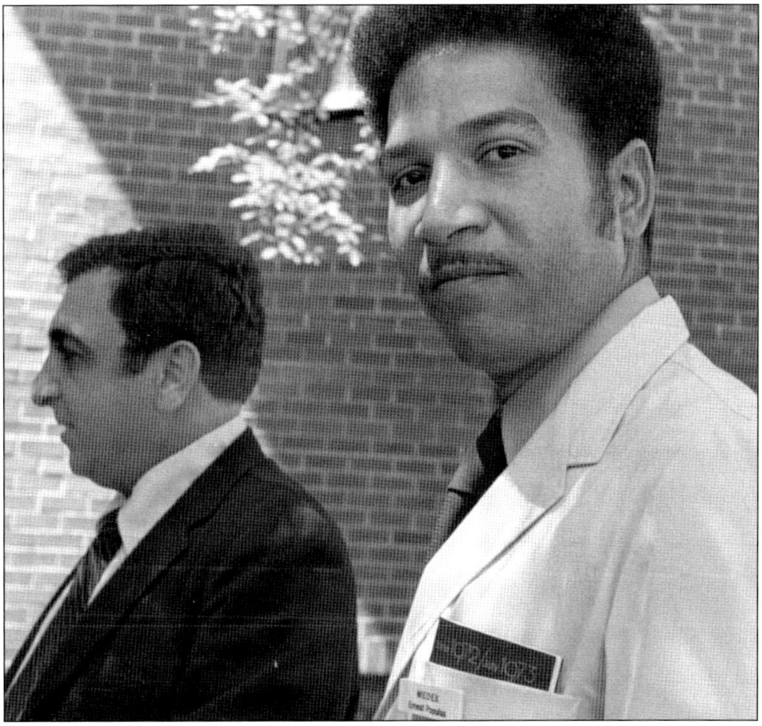

Seattle Urban Practice. Medex Ernest Populus (Class 2) became a leader in working with Seattle's urban population. Populus (right) is seen with MEDEX program administrator Mark Markarian.

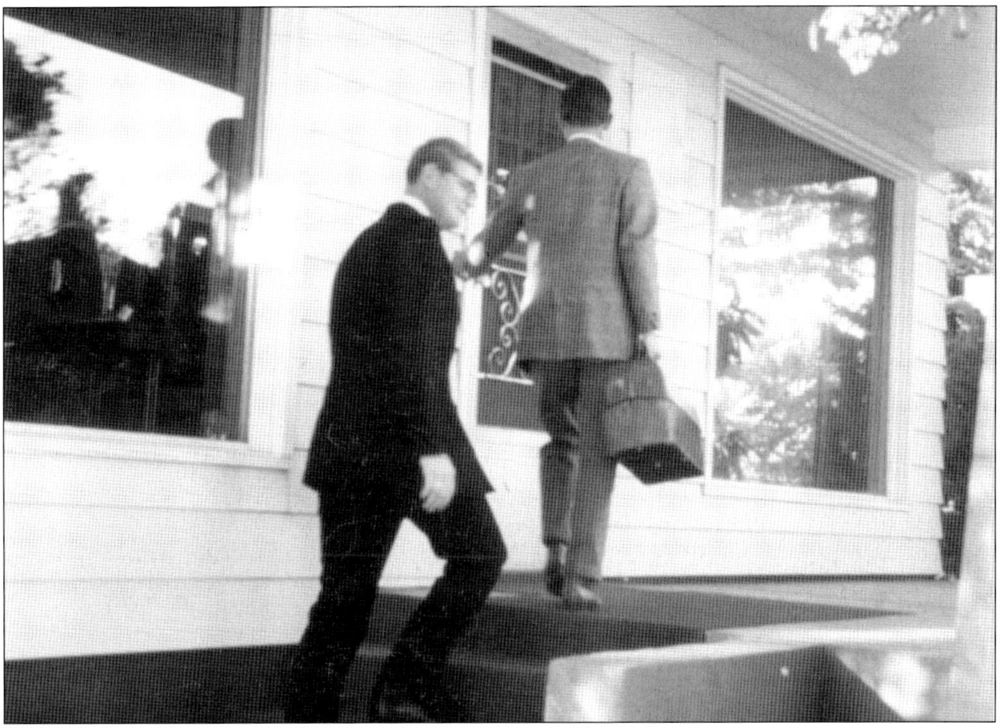

Primary-Care House Calls. In addition to clinic and hospital practice, MEDEX encouraged comprehensive medical care, including house calls. Here, Dean Meade (Class 1, left) is seen with his preceptor G. Dean Barth, MD, visiting a patient at home.

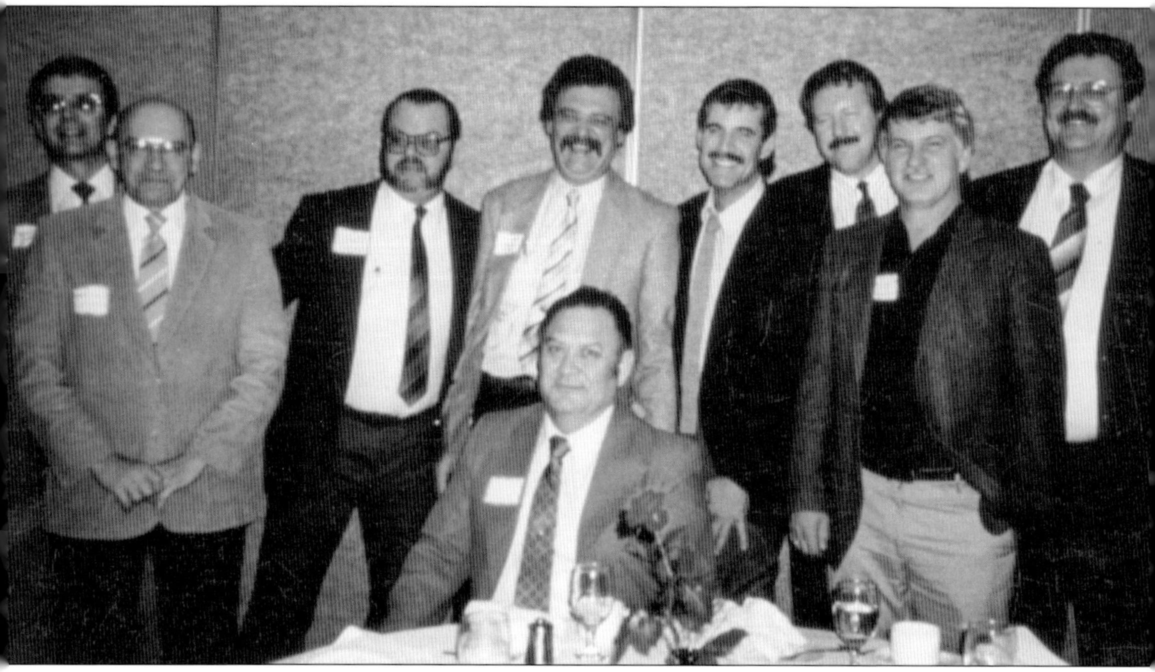

CLASS 1, 20 YEARS LATER. Members of Class 1 are shown at the MEDEX 20th reunion. Many of the group were still in practice—some in their original training/employment sites. They all felt proud to have been the pioneers for MEDEX and role models for many subsequent PA students.

Three

Curriculum Design and Adaptation

As the MEDEX collaborative model of PA education was successfully implemented in Washington State, the founders had bigger aspirations. If this model could improve health-care access in one state with one medical school, why could it not work across the United States? As a "systems thinker," Dr. Richard Smith was interested in the replicability of the MEDEX model. He was aware of Dr. Eugene Stead and the Duke University model (developing the PA profession within a large academic medical center). But for MEDEX, Smith envisioned a markedly different mission, which was rural and primary-care training. He was sure that other medical schools might feel the same way.

Dr. Smith and his expanding set of colleagues aimed for a more generalist training approach, with links to specific communities and populations. Key features of the MEDEX model included considerations of how military corpsmen, as PA students, differed from medical students. This led to the creation of a competency-based curriculum working backward from a needs assessment of the skills that these new professionals would need to have, designing community-based experiences to connect with patients, and focusing on primary care/generalist education that was applicable in both urban and rural settings.

His goal was to have at least one MEDEX program in each US time zone. As a result, the MEDEX network grew to include seven additional medical schools.

Dr. Smith—again based on his Peace Corps experience—actively marketed the new profession. Along with the Duke program, MEDEX was mentioned in the comic strip *Gasoline Alley* where a main character, Chipper Wallet, becomes a PA. Dr. Smith and other PA program founders worked to have PAs included in a wide range of publications, including medical journals, federal reports, and consumer directed publications, like the largest circulating weekly magazine, which was included in most local Sunday newspapers, *Parade*.

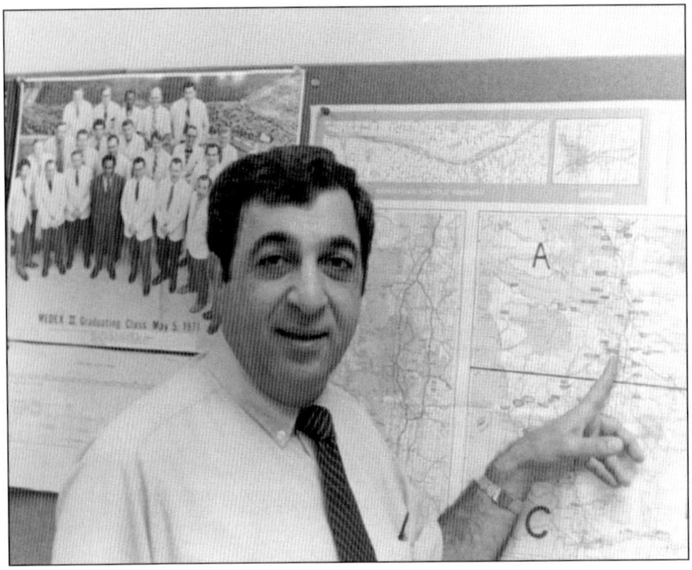

MEDEX NATIONWIDE MAP. MEDEX program administrator Mark Markarian is seen with maps of rural and urban Washington. Soon, the MEDEX concept grew to encompass eight institutions throughout the United States in a group of regional programs designed to collaborate with physicians and communities to train and employ returning military corpsmen. The goal was to have at least one MEDEX program in each continental US time zone.

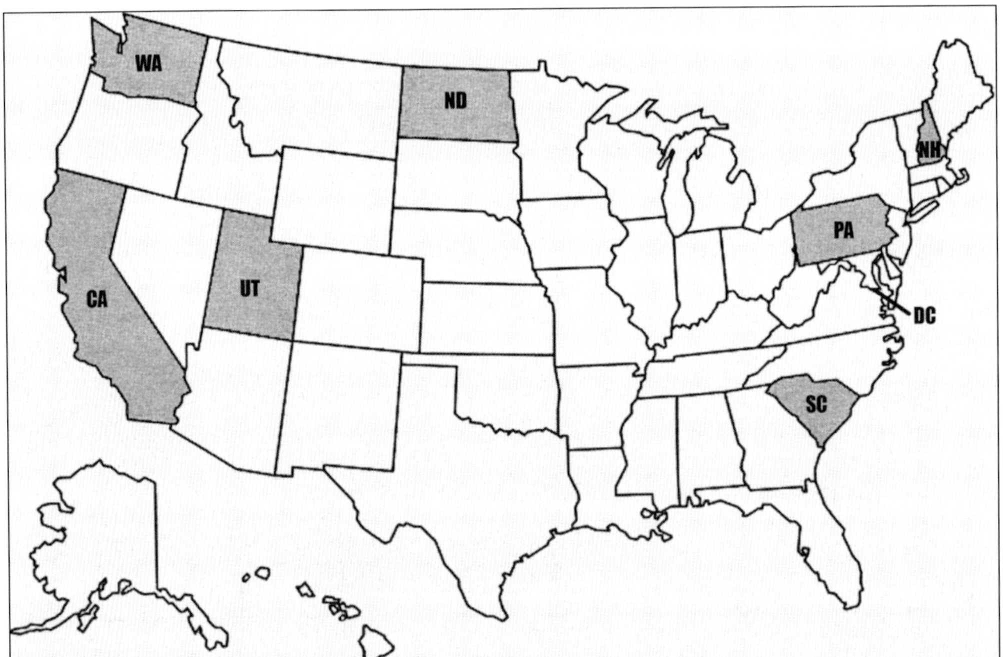

GROWTH OF A DREAM. In the 1970s, Dr. Smith's office map (recreated here) tracked his vision of a MEDEX program in all four time zones: at the University of Washington (Seattle, Washington); Dartmouth College (Hanover, New Hampshire); Howard University (Washington, DC); Charles R. Drew University of Medicine and Science (Los Angeles, California); the University of North Dakota (Grand Forks, North Dakota); the Medical University of South Carolina (Charleston, South Carolina); Pennsylvania State University (Hershey, Pennsylvania); and the University of Utah (Salt Lake City, Utah).

North Dakota Visionary. The North Dakota program was founded by Dr. Robert C. Eelkema, with Judy DeMers and Mickey Knutson serving as faculty and leaders. Dr. Eelkema later published *Medicine in the Back of Beyond*; the book is about how he helped to "pioneer a radical strategy that extended the reach of doctors into rural America." The back cover, pictured here, shows a positive review from Dr. Smith. (Courtesy of Robert C. Eelkema.)

Medicine in the Back of Beyond

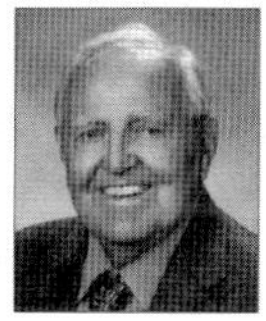

Medicine in the Back of Beyond describes the early and serendipitous opportunities that led to the birth of the MEDEX Program at the University of North Dakota, and how the UND Nurse Practitioner/Physician Assistant Program grew from it.

Part autobiography, part history lesson, Dr. Robert C. Eelkema tells the stories of those who went on to make an essential difference in health care services throughout the nation. Dr. Eelkema looks at his roots and shares the wisdom that comes only from introspection later in life.

Praise for the author of "Medicine in the Back of Beyond"

"Bob Eelkema was one of the first champions of an idea that—at the time—was considered radical in the field of medicine: training a new type of professional to address the lack of health care services in rural and underserved areas. His vision and his tenacity in making that vision a reality, exemplifies the spirit of creativity and innovation that has always moved America forward."

—**DICK SMITH, MD, MPH**
Father of the MEDEX Program
Retired Professor, University of Hawaii
School of Public Health, Honolulu, HI

"Dr. Eelkema was one of the first people to appreciate the potential of using skilled non-physicians for the provision of health care. Although this concept found its first application in primary care, mid-level practitioners are now employed in all medical disciplines. Dr. Eelkema helped to create a sea change in medicine in the 1970s. His account will be of interest to everyone in the field of health care."

—**JAMES BROSSEAU, MD, FACP**
Medical Director, Diabetes Center
Altru Health System, Grand Forks, ND

"Dr. Bob Eelkema is a central figure in the building of the modern UND School of Medicine and Health Sciences. It was Bob's leadership, vision, political savvy, and out-and-out tenacity that created a four-year medical school. Along with this, Bob created the Indians into Medicine Program, the Physician Assistant Program, the original Area Health Education Center that was so pivotal in establishing the four medical school campuses, and the Center for Rural Health which is recognized as a national leader in rural health. Bob's skills may only be matched by his compassion for others and amazing, if not ribald, sense of humor. Many elements of today's medical school would not exist if it were not for Dr. Bob Eelkema."

—**BRAD GIBBENS**
Deputy Director, Center for Rural Health
University of North Dakota School of Medicine and Health Sciences, Grand Forks, ND

ISBN 978-0-9854734-0-2

51995>

9 780985 473402

COVER ILLUSTRATION © CORBIS IMAGES
BACK COVER PHOTO BY BRIAN'S PHOTOGRAPHY
COVER DESIGN BY GARY NIEMEIER

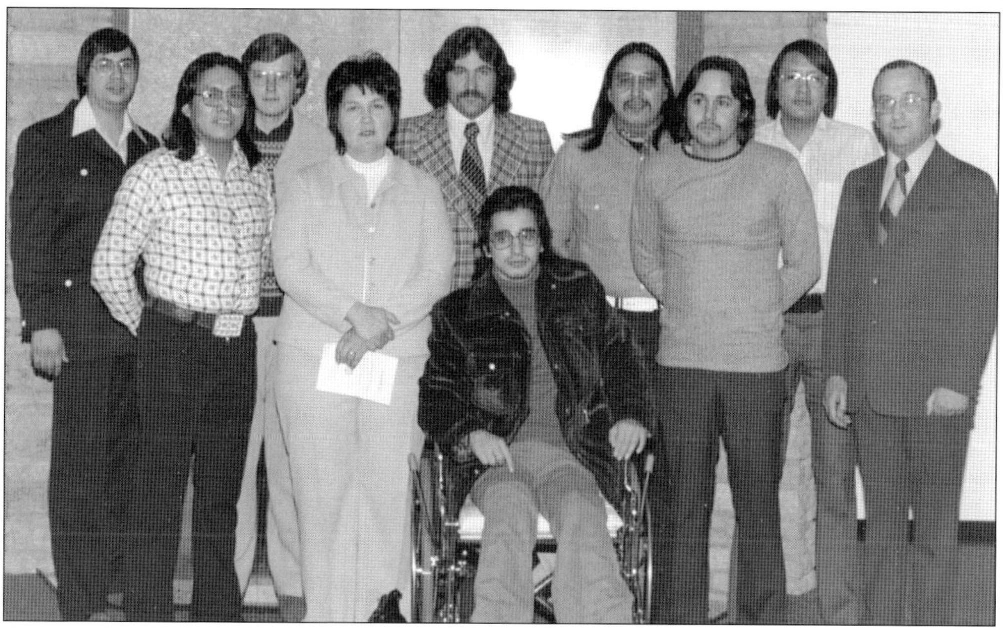

North Dakota Graduating Class. The University of North Dakota placed special emphasis on recruiting class members from reservations and small communities in the Dakotas. Shown here are members of the third graduating class in 1975; from left to right are (first row) Robert Stands, Thalma Selwyn, James Iron Shell, Robert Lieberman, and Richard Schlosser; (second row) Timothy Yellow, Steven Fandre, Robert Cox, Floyd Oliver, and Fred Brings Him Back. (Courtesy of University of North Dakota PA program.)

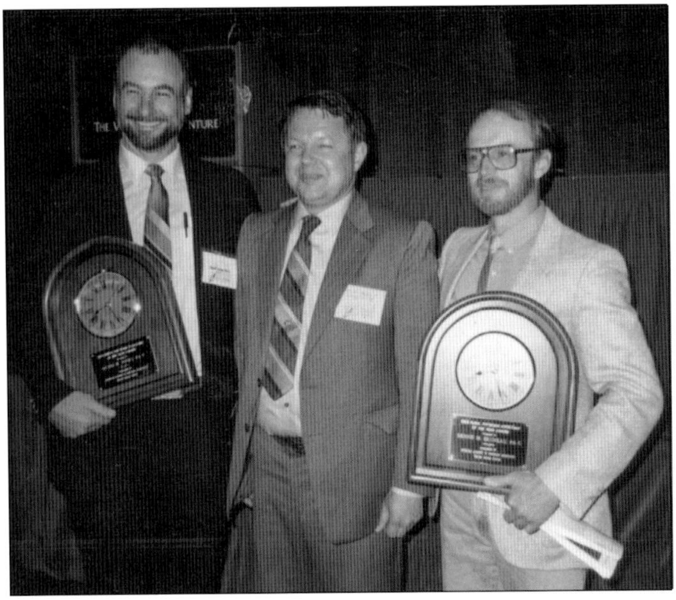

NORTH DAKOTA INNOVATION. North Dakota graduates influenced care in many rural communities. Pictured here are David Jones (Class 9, left) and Dennis Bruneau, a North Dakota graduate (right) with their supervising physician in Condon, Oregon. In 1988, they received the Rural PA Award from the American Academy of Physician Assistants. Bruneau and Jones also served on the MEDEX faculty. (Courtesy of Physician Assistant History Society, Johns Creek, Georgia.)

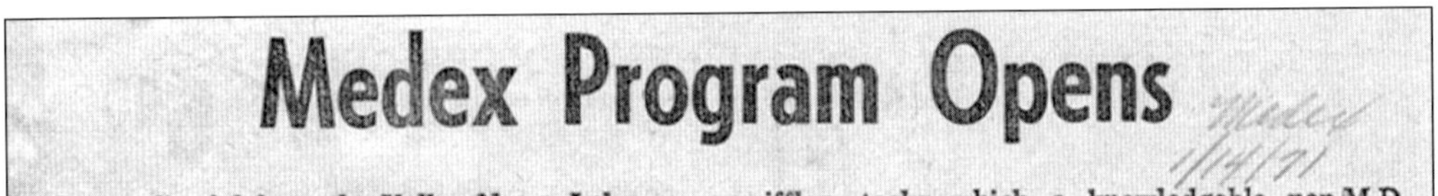

Medex Program Opens

Guest editorial from the Valley News, Lebanon.

* * *

The Medex program which began this week at Dartmouth Medical School is an important step toward easing the acute shortage of health care providers in Northern New England.

The program will provide extensive training to young people who already have considerable background in medical care, obtained in many cases in the armed forces.

Medex training will provide them with more skills and education so that they'll be able to work successfully as assistants to practicing physicians.

The aim of the Medex concept is based on the contention that many, if not most, general practitioners spend a large amount of their valuable time doing work that could easily be handled by trained assistants. One such area, for example, is well-baby care, where many physicians now devote much time to such chores as weighing infants and counselling mothers on care of sniffles, tasks which a knowledgable non-M.D. helper could handle.

Rural Northern New England and many other parts of the nation are generally deficient in good health care services. By freeing the available physicians of menial work, better disease prevention and treatment will be provided to many more people.

Perhaps the biggest problem the Medex program will encounter will be reluctance on the part of some patients to be treated by a paraprofessional rather than a physician. But such fears are groundless so long as the physician supervises the Medex assistant as the program intends.

Anyone who has served in the armed forces knows that paraprofessionals handle a substantial share of the medical care work for both uniformed and dependent personnel.

The Dartmouth Medex program is a significant step toward better health and a better life for North New England residents.

DARTMOUTH ANNOUNCING MEDEX. This January 1971 clipping from the *Manchester Union-Leader* describes the opening of the Dartmouth MEDEX program, dedicated to serving rural communities of Northern New England. The students and graduates were carefully studied by Dartmouth researchers with regard to patient acceptance and the level of tasks assigned by physicians. (Courtesy of Rauner Special Collections, Dartmouth University.)

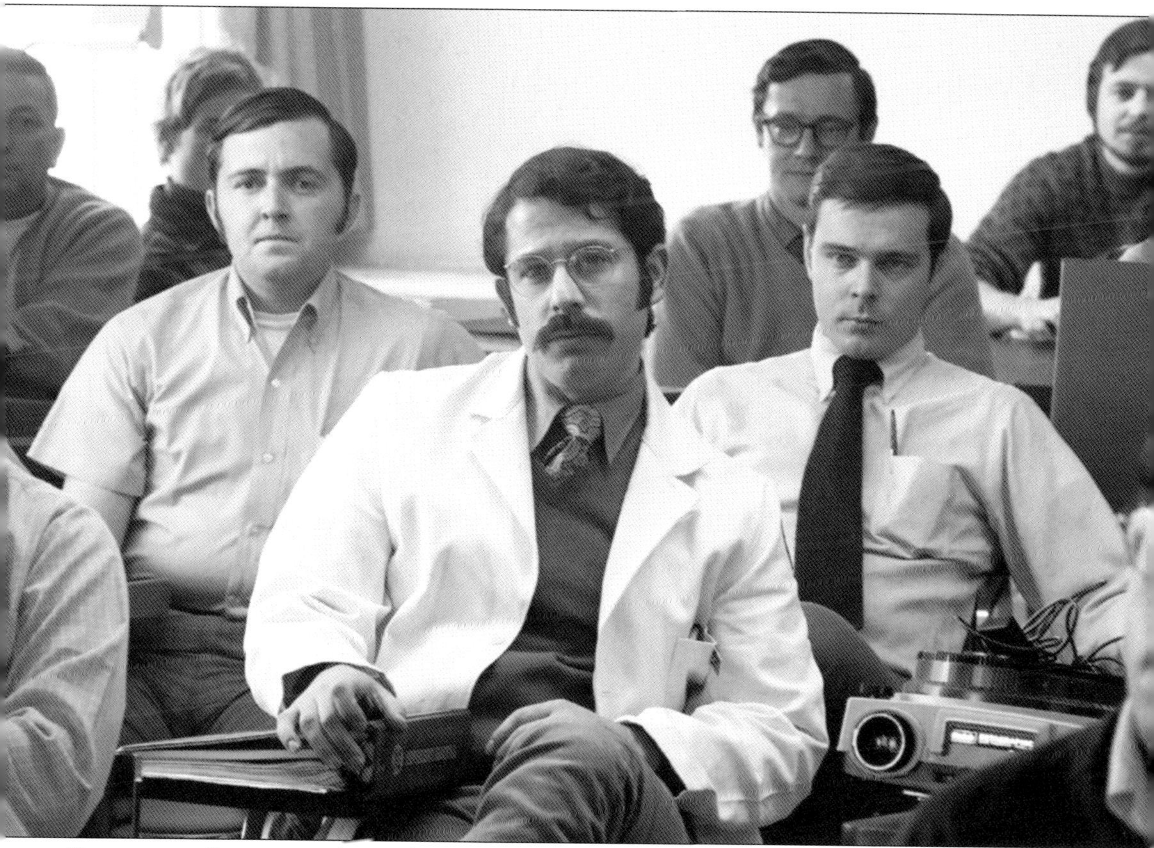

DARTMOUTH CLASSROOM. As in other early Physician Assistant programs, students in the Dartmouth MEDEX program were all males with extensive prior medical backgrounds, usually in the military. These Dartmouth students are pictured in a classroom on campus. The early MEDEX curriculum model included three months of classroom placements followed by 15 to 18 months of clinical experiences in rural family medicine practices where the physicians had agreed to hire them upon graduation. (Courtesy of Rauner Special Collections, Dartmouth University.)

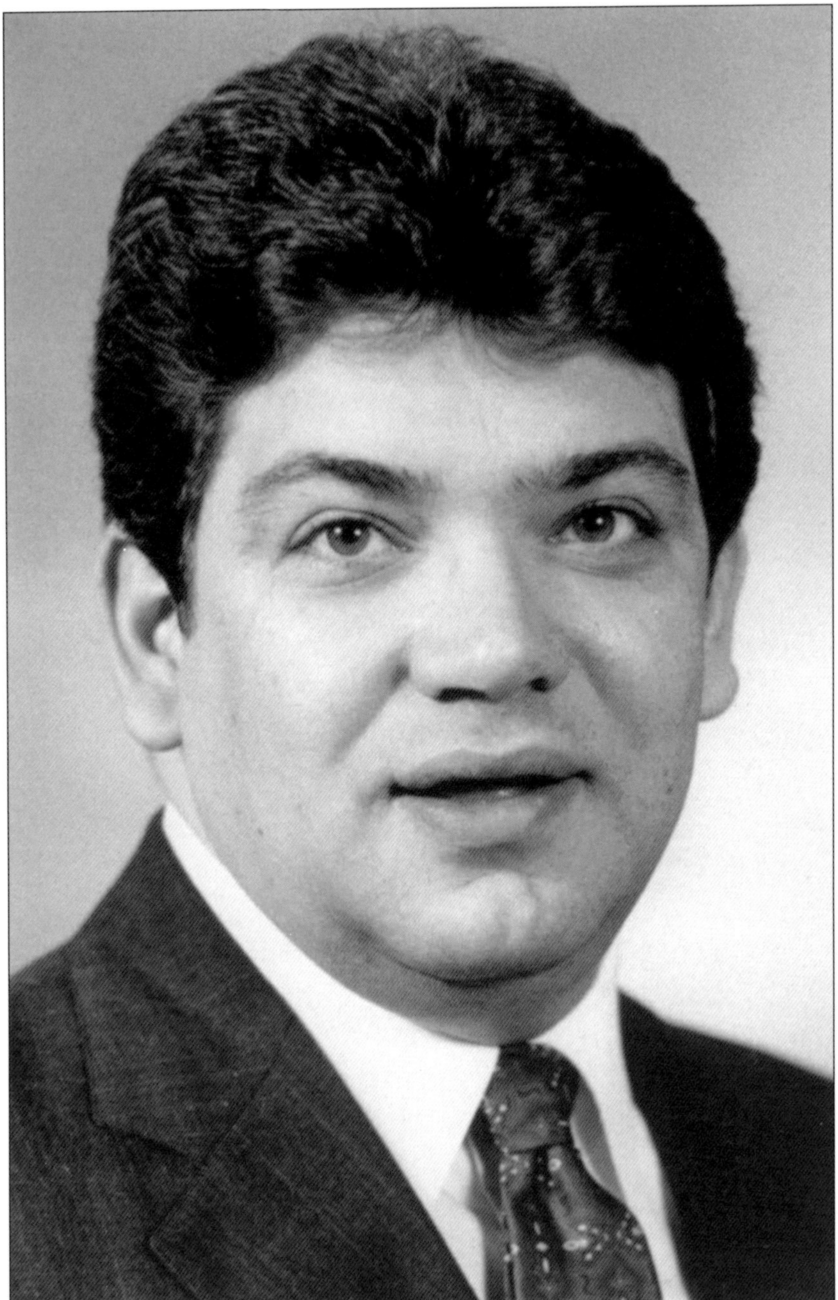

PA Leader from the Dartmouth Program. R. Scott Chavez, PA-C, PhD, a distinguished graduate of the Dartmouth Physician Assistant Program in 1974, served in the US Air Force from 1967 to 1973. Scott practiced in California, Arizona, Nevada, and Nebraska. He served as president of the AAPA in 1987 and served as the AAPA liaison to the AMA from 1988 to 1987. He taught at the University of Nebraska and was founding chair for the Midwestern University Physician Assistant Program at Downers Grove. He was a leading authority on US correctional health systems, serving as vice president and director of accreditation for the National Commission on Correctional Health Care. (Courtesy of Physician Assistant History Society, Johns Creek, Georgia.)

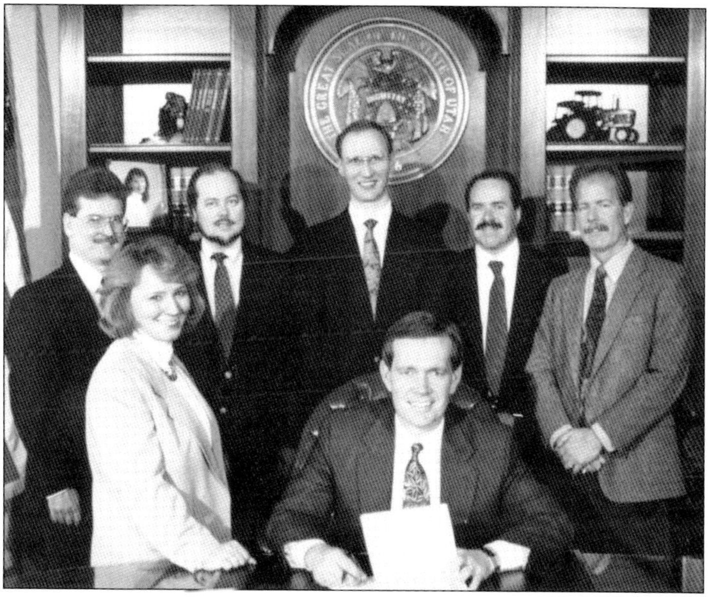

Utah PA Bill. Utah governor Michael Leavitt signs a bill expanding PA practice in Utah. Standing in front is Rep. Christine Fox. In the back row are, from left to right, three members from the Department of Health, including Robert Sherwood behind the governor; Bruce Callister, PA-C (then president of the Utah Academy of PAs); and Donald M. Pedersen, PhD., PA, of the Utah Physician Assistant Program, now clinical professor emeritus.

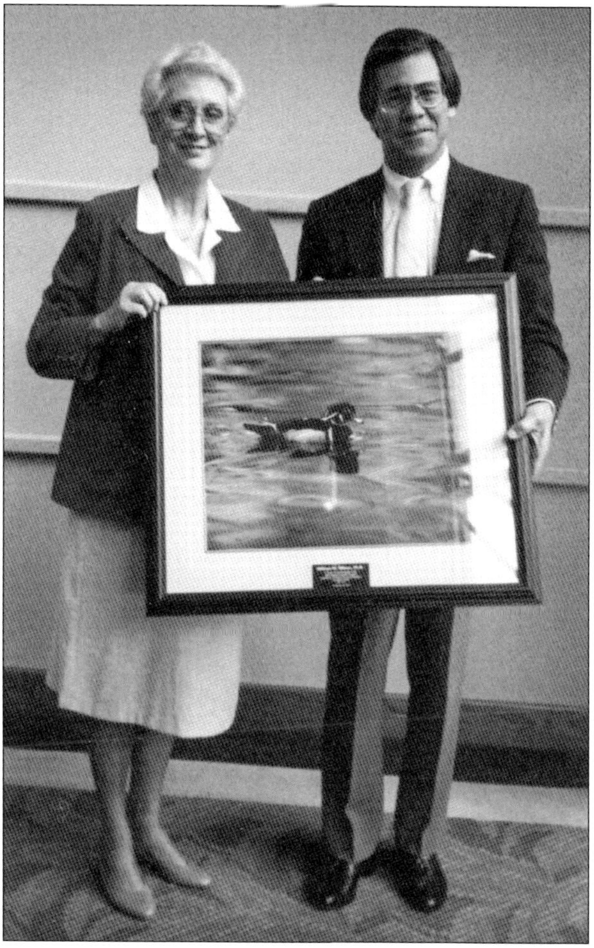

Bishop and Wilson. Marian Bishop, PhD, chair of the Department of Family and Preventive Medicine at the University of Utah, is shown with Bill Wilson, Utah MEDEX founding program director and cofounder of the University of Utah MEDEX Physician Assistant Program. "Bill was a pioneer," said Don Pedersen in his eulogy for Wilson. "He, along with other like-minded individuals in the late 1960s and early 1970s charted the course of a grand social experiment—The Physician Assistant Profession." (Courtesy of University of Utah PA Program.)

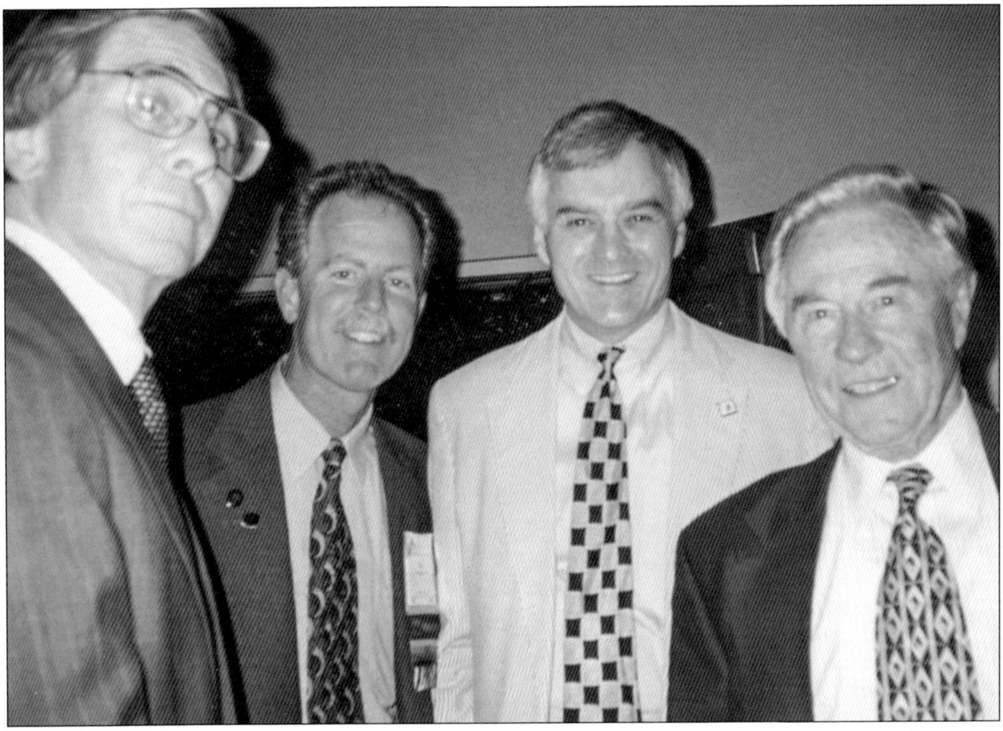

Utah Program Leaders. From left to right, program director Bill Wilson, faculty members Don Pedersen and George White, and medical director Hilmon Castle attend a Utah PA program Event in the 1980s. (Courtesy of University of Utah PA Program.)

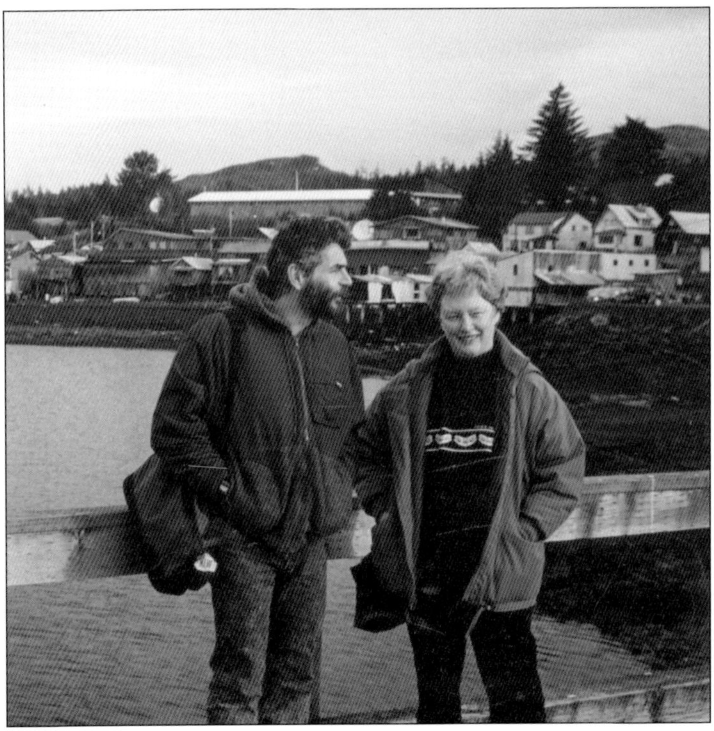

Harry Felton's Contributions. Utah Class 1 graduate Harry Felton had a far-reaching impact on the PA profession as one of the first PAs to serve in a faculty role. Felton was known for his lively teaching style, his concern for rural communities, and his support of military veterans. He later practiced in Kodiak, and then Sitka, Alaska, where he helped to establish the first MEDEX Alaska training site. He is shown here with MEDEX director Ruth Ballweg visiting the clinic in Kake, Alaska.

Charles R. Drew PA Program. Dr. M. Alfred Haines, MD, served as the founder of the Charles R. Drew Physician Assistant Program. Physician assistant Ruth Webb served as program director beginning in 1973. Unfortunately, there were no photographs of these two leaders available of sufficient quality. Pictured is Steve Turnipseed (Class 1), consultant for the Drew program regarding the MEDEX model of PA training. (Courtesy of Group Health Cooperative Archives.)

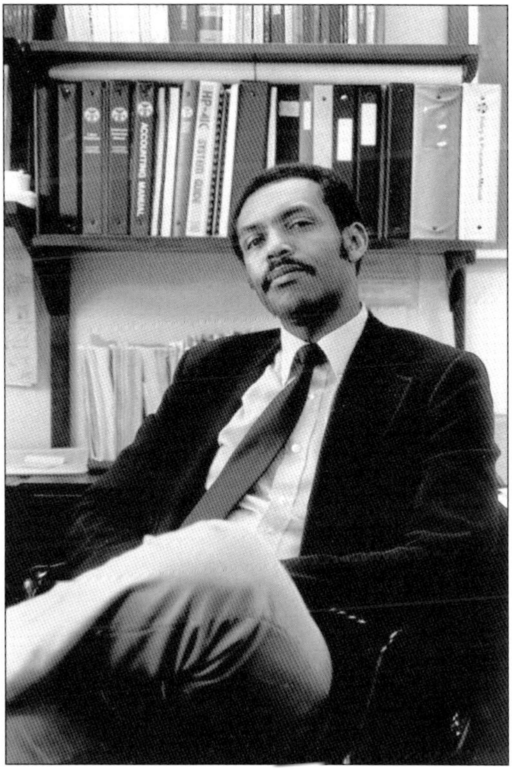

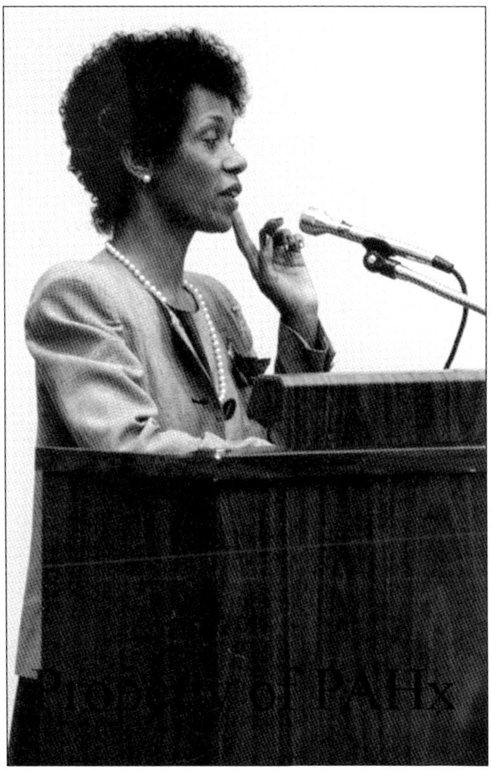

Drew Graduate Becoming a Leader. Drew graduate Brenda Jasper, PA-C, was director of the Howard PA program for years. She was vice president of APAP (one of the first African Americans in APAP leadership) and was a driving force behind the creation of Project Access and the AAPA African Heritage Caucus. She was the founding director of the PA program at the University of Maryland Eastern Shore and a clinician with the Department of Veterans Affairs. (Courtesy of Physician Assistant History Society, Johns Creek, Georgia.)

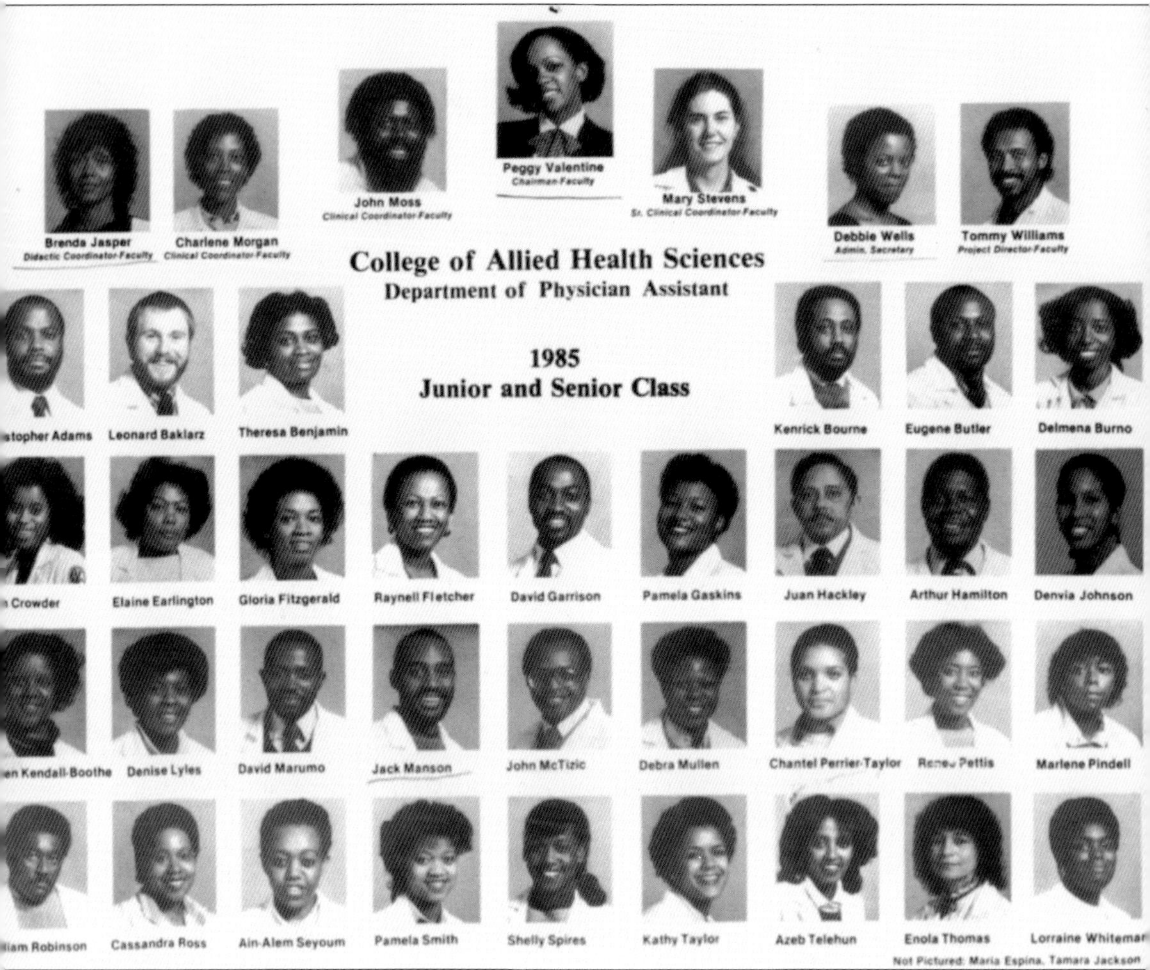

Howard University Program. This is the only photograph obtained from the early Howard program, founded in 1974. But this book would be incomplete without some visual tribute to this prominent teaching institution for minority PAs nationwide. In the words of current director Shelly Powers (shown here as student Shelly Spires), "Over one-third of the nation's practicing African American PAs are Howard graduates." (Courtesy of Howard University.)

Four

Progress at the State and National Level

To develop and thrive, the emerging PA profession would need the support of the medical establishment. From the beginning, the Washington State Medical Association (WSMA) became an extremely supportive ally, in partnership with the relatively new University of Washington School of Medicine. They have remained strong supporters through the years. In 1971, the WSMA sponsored its first bill in the state legislature—the PA licensing law, Revised Code of Washington, Chapter 18.71A. It was designed to support physicians and to increase health-care access. The legislation was introduced by Dr. Jim McDermott, a physician serving in the Washington state legislature, now a senior US congressman from Washington's 7th District who continues to support PA initiatives at the federal level.

Passage of the law was supported by veterans' associations in Washington State; busloads of veterans converged on the state capitol in Olympia to urge support of the bill. Over time, the bill has been modified and expanded to reflect current physician/physician assistant practice. As the result of legislative action supported by the WSMA, two PAs now serve on the Washington medical board—the Medical Quality Assurance Commission. The Washington Academy of Physician Assistants also has a seat in the WSMA House of Delegates, and PAs also serve on the WSMA Interspecialty Council.

Nationally, there was growing collaboration between representatives of the educational models created at Duke University (Physician Assistant), the University of Washington (Medex), the University of Colorado (Child Health Associate), Alderson Broaddus College (Baccalaureate), and the University of Alabama at Birmingham (PA Surgeon Assistant). Professional PAs joined ranks within the existing American Academy of Physician Assistants. Similarly, program directors joined ranks to form the Association of Physician Assistant Programs, now the Physician Assistant Education Association. A landmark national conference sponsored jointly by these two organizations was held in Wichita Falls, Texas, in 1973. The next steps were the creation of an accreditation body—the Joint Review Committee (JRC-PA), now the Accreditation Review Commission (ARC-PA) and a certification organization, the National Commission on Certification of Physician Assistants (NCCPA).

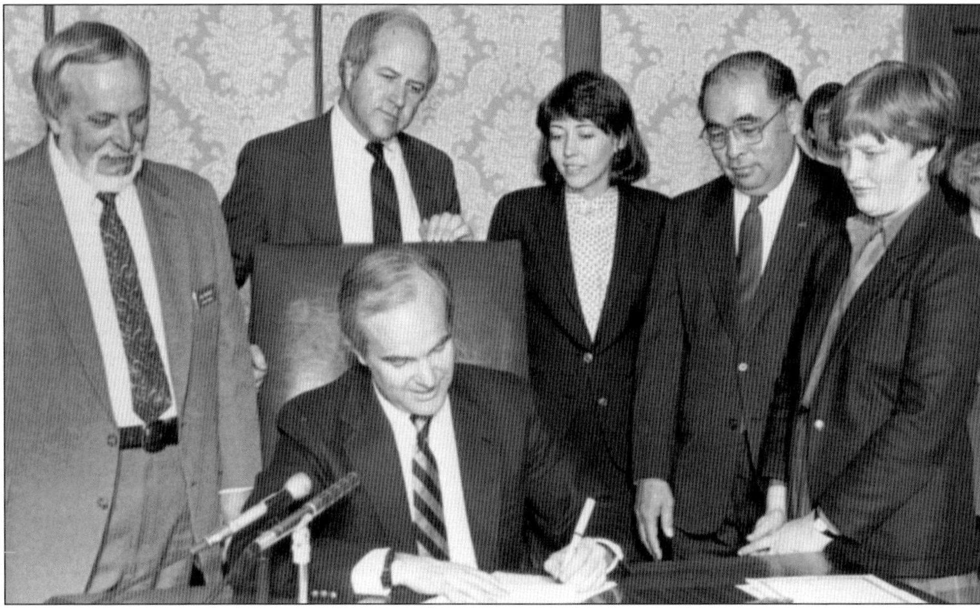

Signing of PA Legislation. Since the initial Washington State PA Licensing Act in 1971, other legislation has supported expanded practice. Gov. Dan Evans is shown in 1987 signing legislation that added a PA to the Washington Medical Quality Assurance Commission. Maria Cantwell was the sponsor of the bill during her first term in the state legislature. Two lobbyists from WSMA are standing first and second from left with now senator Cantwell standing at center. WAPA president Shinobu Inouye stands beside MEDEX director Ruth Ballweg at far right. (Author's collection.)

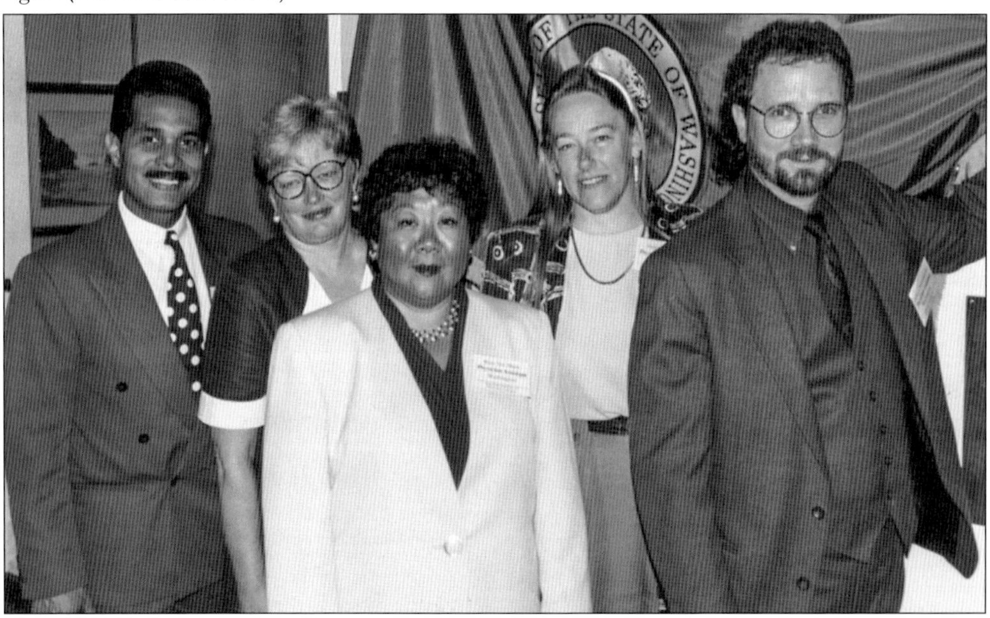

WAPA Lobbying in Washington, DC. MEDEX graduates representing the Washington Academy of Physician Assistants have participated in annual AAPA lobbying experiences in Washington, DC. This group included Ed Lopez (Class 15), Ruth Ballweg (Class 11), Wen-Yee Shaw (Class 26), Helen Hancken (Class 24), and Jim Cherewatenko, president of WAPA. (Author's collection.)

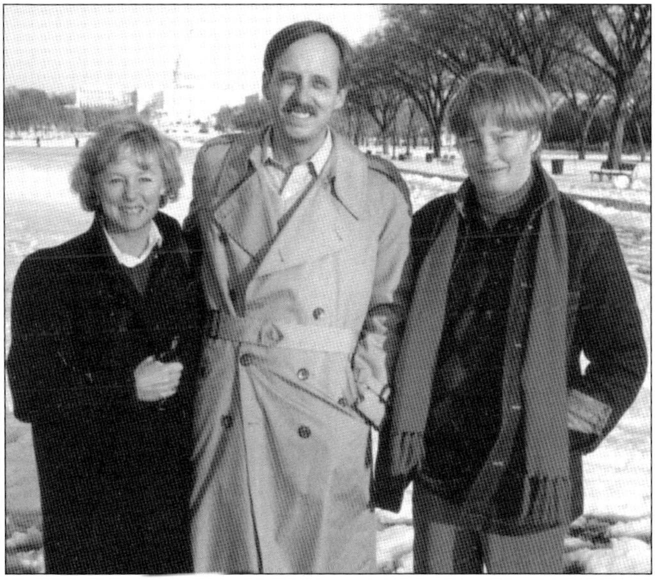

MEDEX Lobbying in Washington, DC. MEDEX leaders also participated in Washington, DC, lobbying in activities organized by the Association of Physician Assistant Programs (now the Physician Assistant Education Association). From left to right, program administrator Jennifer Johnston, associate director Henry Stoll, and program director Ruth Ballweg are seen on the snowy Washington Mall in 1989. (Author's collection.)

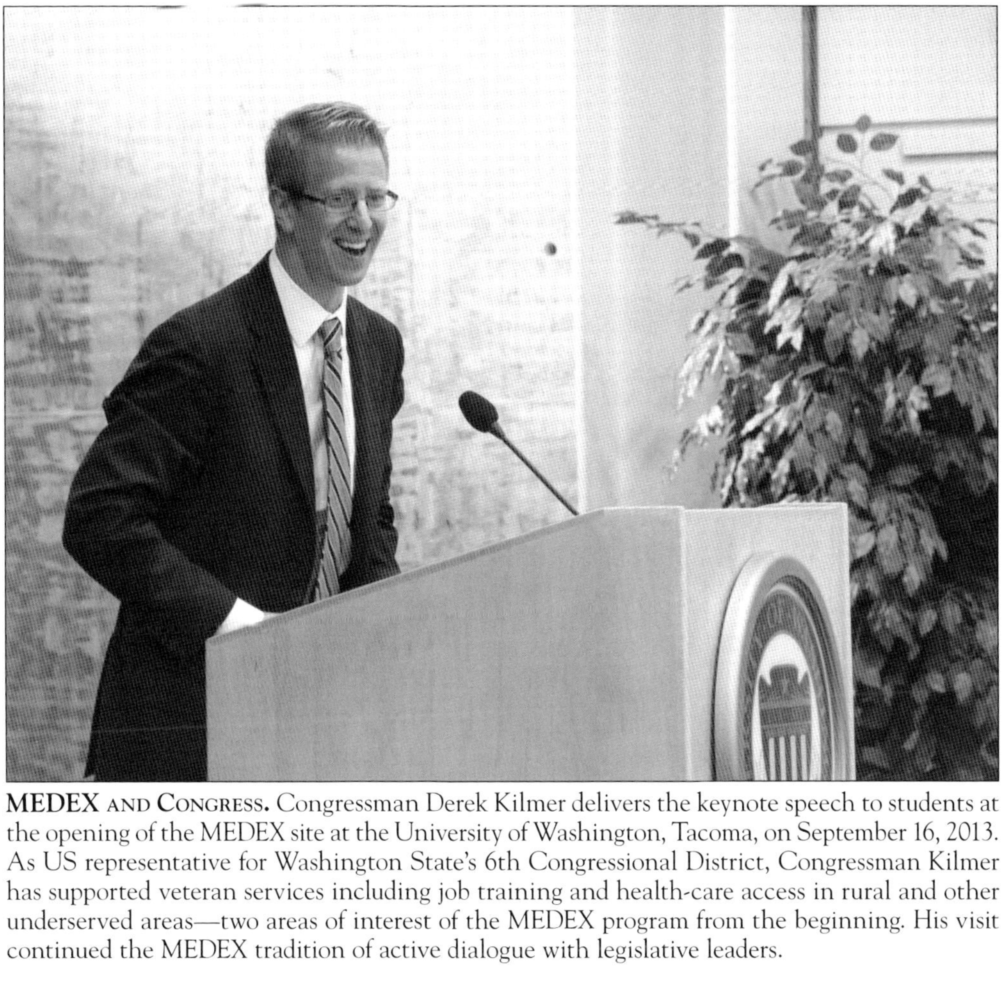

MEDEX and Congress. Congressman Derek Kilmer delivers the keynote speech to students at the opening of the MEDEX site at the University of Washington, Tacoma, on September 16, 2013. As US representative for Washington State's 6th Congressional District, Congressman Kilmer has supported veteran services including job training and health-care access in rural and other underserved areas—two areas of interest of the MEDEX program from the beginning. His visit continued the MEDEX tradition of active dialogue with legislative leaders.

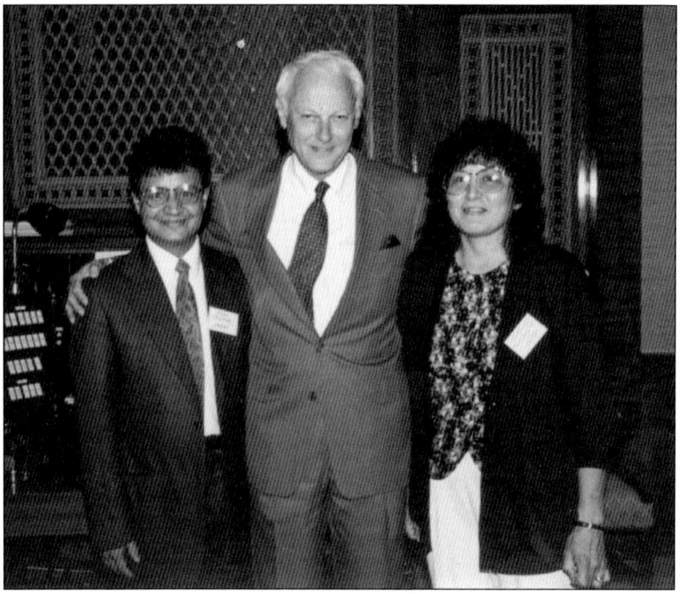

University of Washington Presidential Reception. Hosting an annual reception for students, University of Washington president William Gerberding (center) is pictured with Ram Sharma (Class Part-Time 5, left) and Sonia Vent (Class 17).

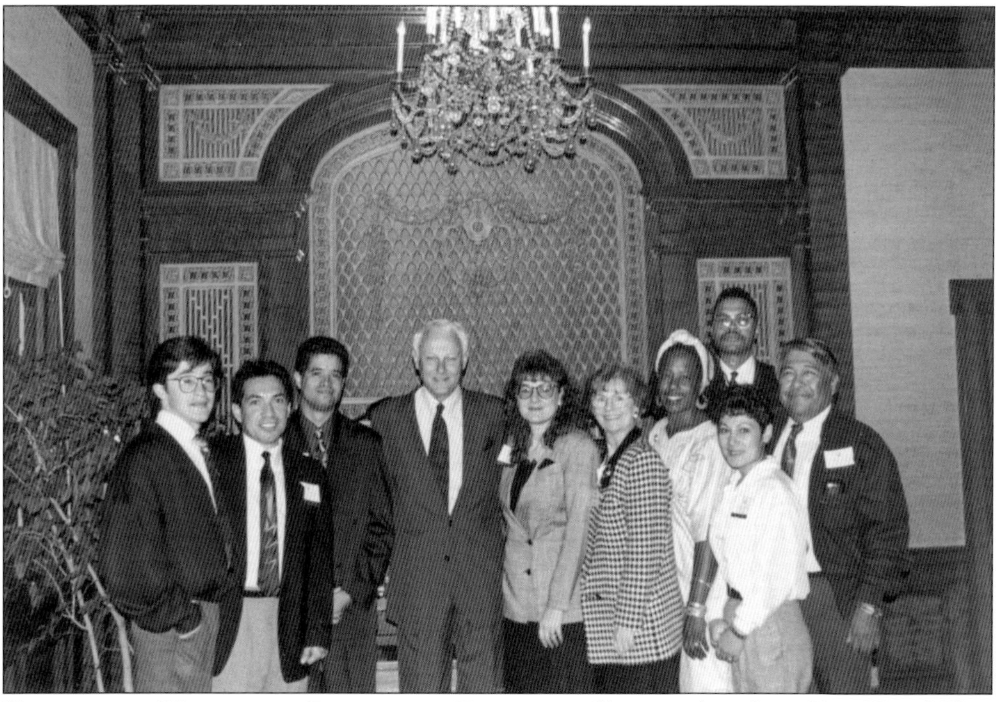

University of Washington Presidential Reception. Class members from Class 27 and Class Part-Time 4 are pictured with University of Washington president William Gerberding. From left to right are Elmer Sisneros, Armando Garcia, Hector Gutierrez Jr., William Gerberding, Laurie Benton, Doreen Blomstrand (faculty), Pamela Asadi, William Shawn Lax (back), Shirley Haynes (front), and Lancelot Lewis.

LEGACY OF LEADERS. Dr. Smith provided students with strong leadership role models. In addition, he empowered students with skills and connections to assume leadership at the workplace, community, state level, and beyond. At the 1970 meeting of the Washington State Medical Association in Spokane, Smith provides networking support to Eddie Bivens (Class 1). From left to right are Smith, Bivens, WSMA president Dr. Richard Greenleaf, and Sen. Al Henry.

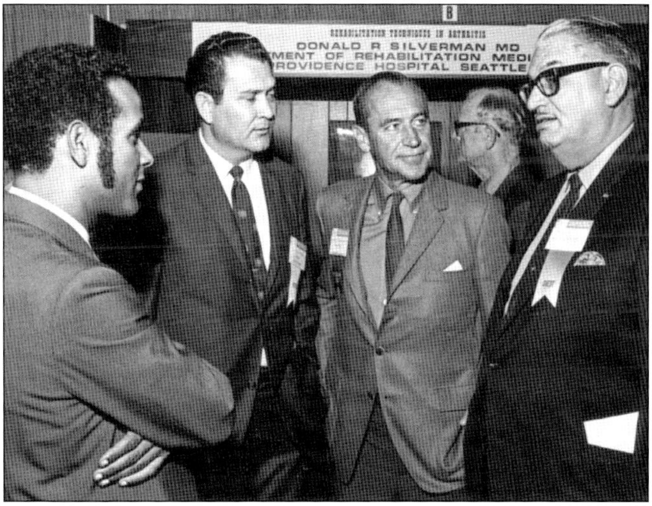

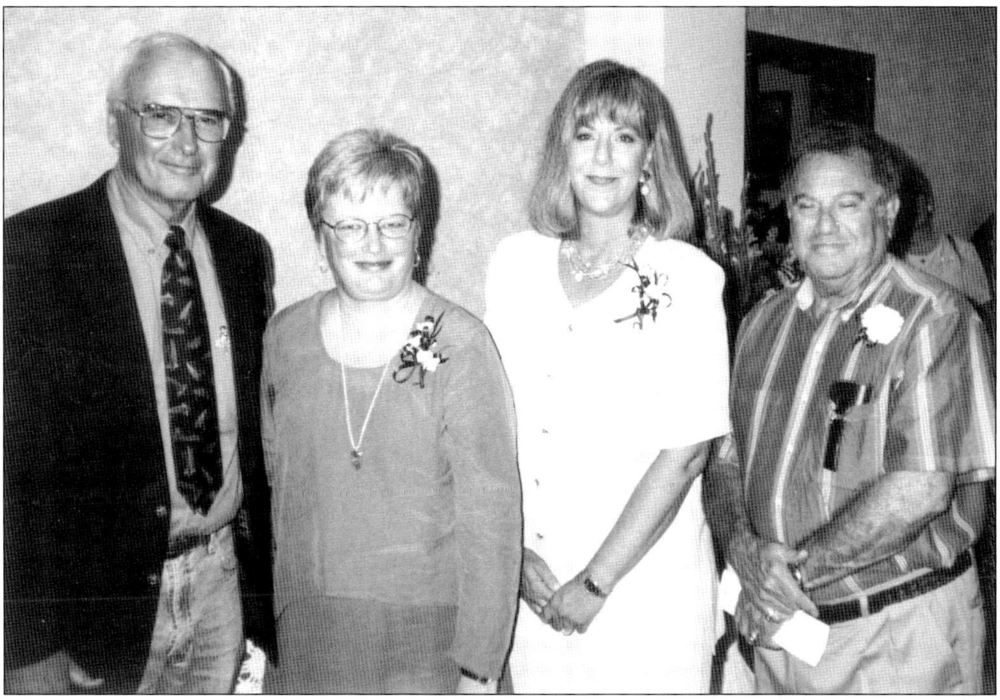

YAKIMA CLASS 1. The Yakima community celebrated the graduation of Yakima Class 1 with a reception that also honored state senator Alex Deccio—the Yakima legislator who was key to receiving state support for MEDEX Eastern Washington Activities. From left to right are Dr. Phil Cleveland, the WWAMI Eastern Washington dean; Ruth Ballweg, MEDEX director; Barbara Gunter-Flynn, MEDEX site director for Yakima; and Senator Deccio.

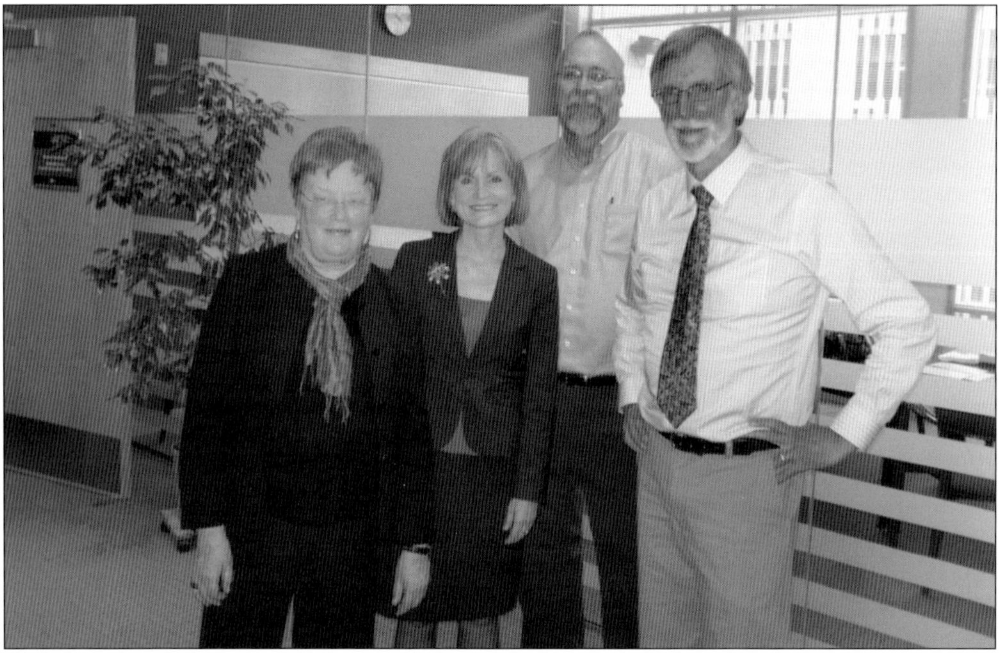

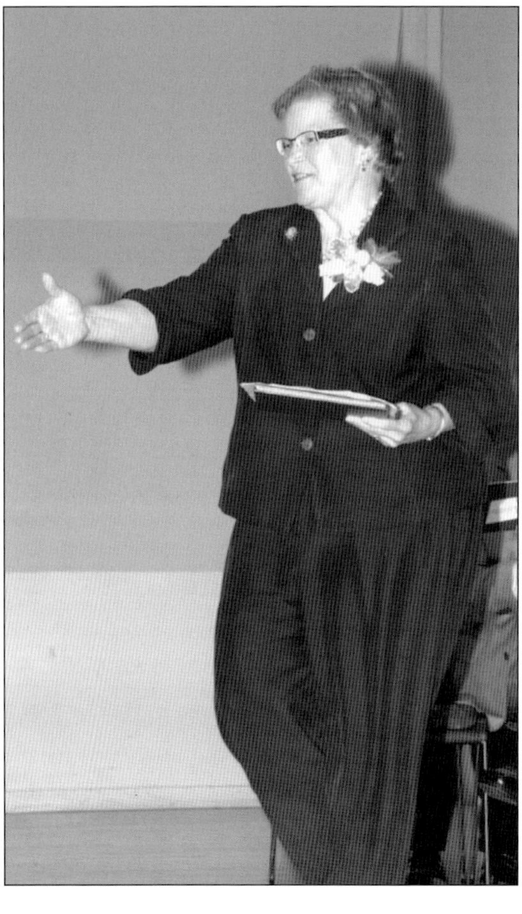

Federal Visitor. Mary Wakefield, administrator of the Federal Health Resources and Services Administration (HRSA), visited MEDEX in 2013 to review strategies for educating returning military medical personnel. She visited with students who talked to her about their experience in MEDEX. From left to right are Ruth Ballweg; Wakefield; Eric Larson, director of the Office of Rural Health Research; and Dr. Louis Fiset, dental director of the DENTEX Dental Therapy program in partnership with the Alaska Native Tribal Health Consortium.

State Public Health Officer. Mary Selecky was Washington state secretary of health for 14 years. In that role, she visited MEDEX to lecture on public health topics and participate in graduations. Selecky is seen presenting a governor's plaque in recognition of physician assistants' contributions to health care in Washington State. As secretary, Selecky was known for her passionate advocacy of public health measures including smoking cessation, improved vaccination rates, patient safety, and preparation for earthquakes, floods, and epidemics.

Five

Adapting MEDEX Over Time

MEDEX has held fast to the values set forth by its founder, Dr. Richard Smith. MEDEX continues to value diversity—in the broadest sense—in its student body and faculty members. The first female students were Patricia Modlin-Rogers (Class 3) and Sue Sanders (Class 6). With Class 7, MEDEX admitted women who were dually enrolled in the School of Nursing and went on to become the school's first nurse practitioners (NPs). In the following year, the NP program formally opened as a separate program in the School of Nursing. Women continued to be enrolled in the MEDEX program in large numbers from then on. In 1974, MEDEX opened its doors to individuals with allied health backgrounds including paramedics, as well as surgical and laboratory technologists. Since the late 1970s, MEDEX classes have been composed of equal numbers of men and women. This equality continues at MEDEX despite the national trend toward classes composed almost exclusively of women. MEDEX has continued to value and welcome returning military medical personnel. One major change has been that now men and women serve as corpsmen and corpswomen in the military service. MEDEX military class members personify that transition.

While maintaining its generalist primary-care focus, the MEDEX curriculum has also expanded and diversified across time to reflect new and broader PA roles. In 1983, the program was expanded to 18 months with additional didactic and clinical coursework. In 1986, the first MEDEX bachelor's degree was awarded. In 1990, the program added a part-time option to allow a limited number of students to continue working during their PA education. In 1992, the curriculum was further expanded to include three additional months of clinical rotations. In 2001, the program added a summer basic science component. In 2004, anatomy and physiology became an online review course taken prior to the basic science courses.

In keeping with the accreditation requirement that all PA programs move to the master's level by 2020, MEDEX transitioned its Seattle and Spokane classes to a master's degree curriculum in 2009, and also created an extended master's degree. Tacoma and Anchorage will gradually move to the master's degree by the required date.

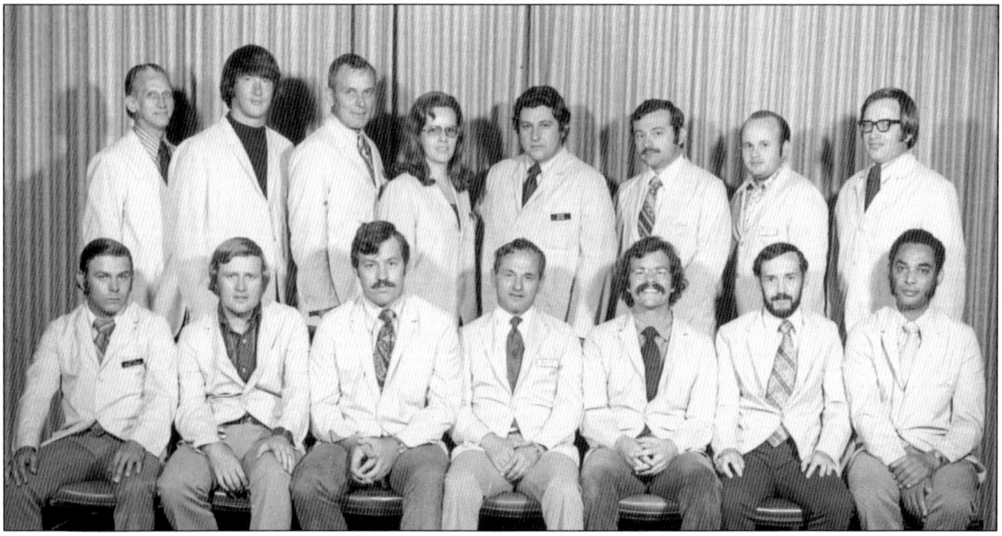

The First Female MEDEX Northwest PA. The first woman student was admitted into MEDEX Class 3 and is seen in the middle of the back row of this photograph of the group. Patricia Modlin-Rogers had similar military training as her male classmates.

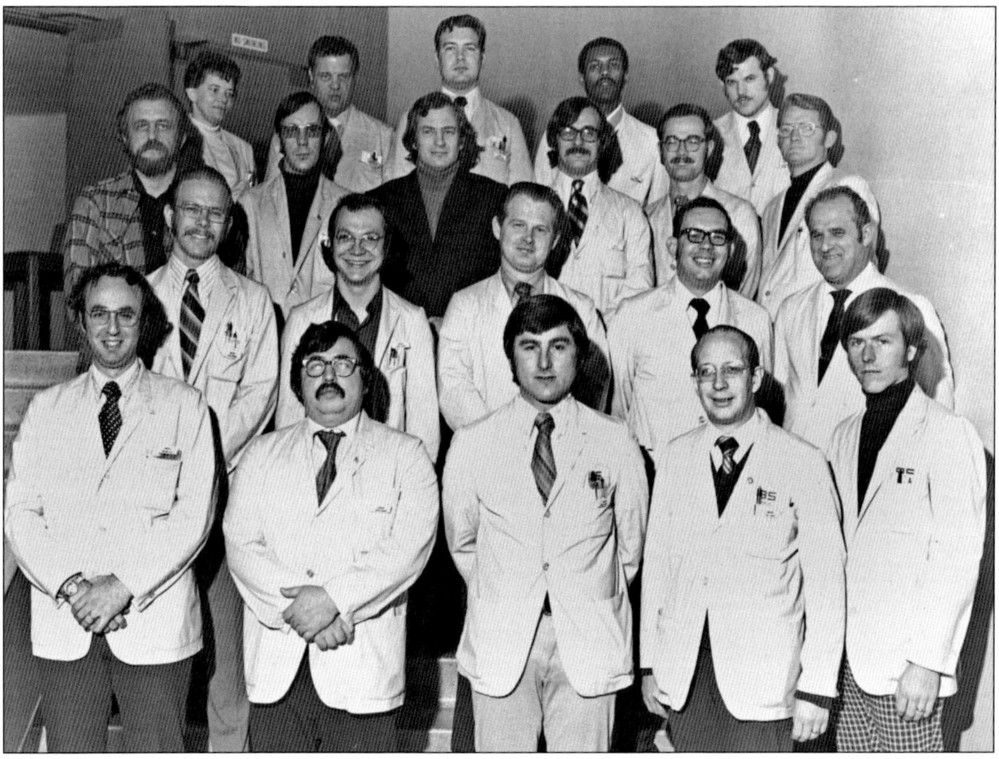

The Second Female MEDEX Northwest PA. The Class 6 MEDEX photograph shows Sue Sanders, the second woman to graduate from MEDEX, at far left in the last row. This photograph also shows Steven Turnipseed (Class 1) as a faculty member. The second MEDEX program director, Dr. David Lawrence, is third from the left in the third row.

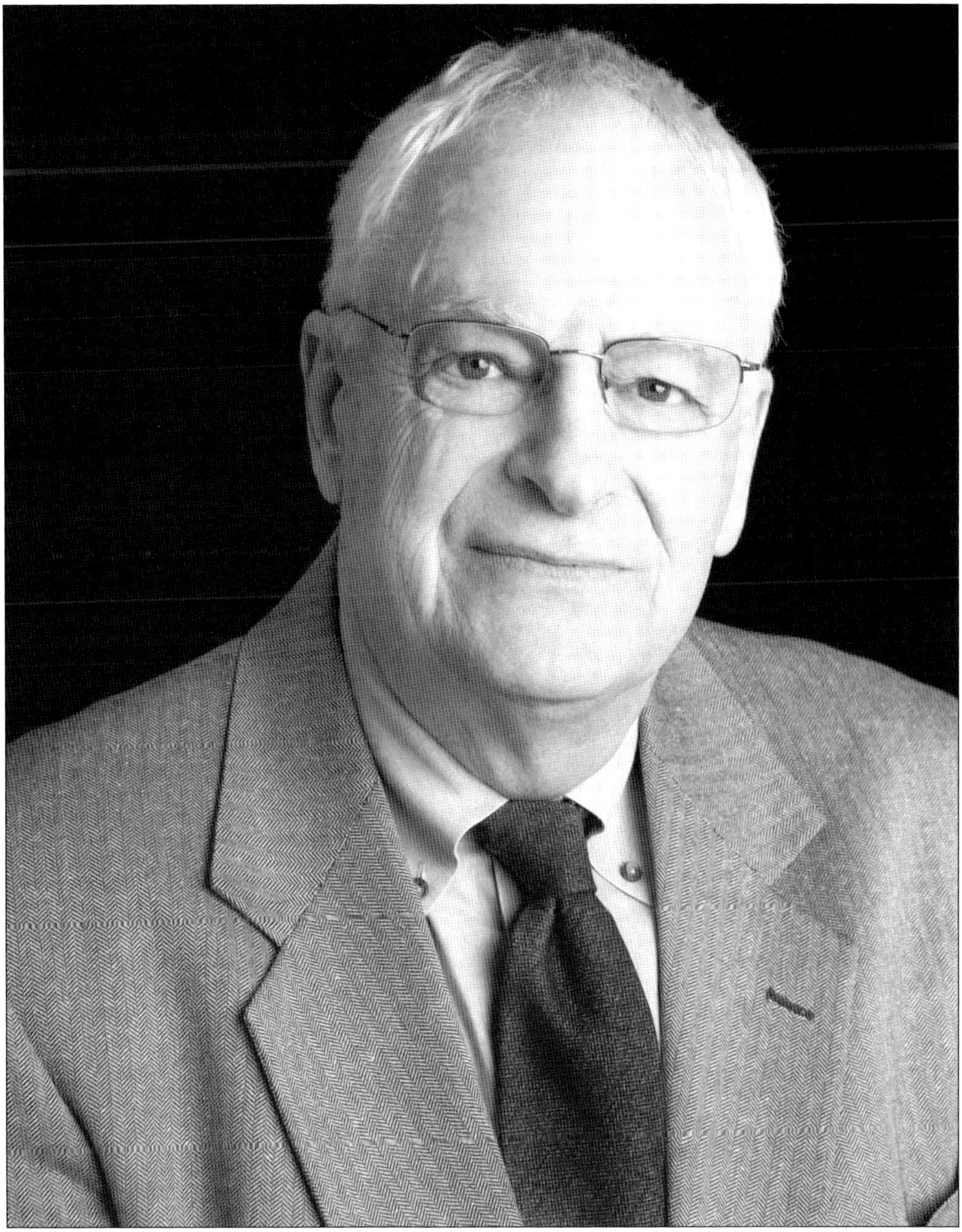

Second Director. Dr. David Lawrence came to the MEDEX program as Dr. Richard Smith moved on to the University of Hawaii. Dr. Lawrence was a Peace Corps physician in the Dominican Republic and advisor to the Ministry of Health in Chile. He then became the "settler" to Dr. Smith's "pioneer." He solidified the program's role within the School of Public Health and built alliances with the School of Nursing. Dr. Lawrence later moved on to many leadership positions, including the CEO and chairman of the board for Kaiser Permanente. (Courtesy of the Physician Assistant History Society Archives, Johns Creek, Georgia.)

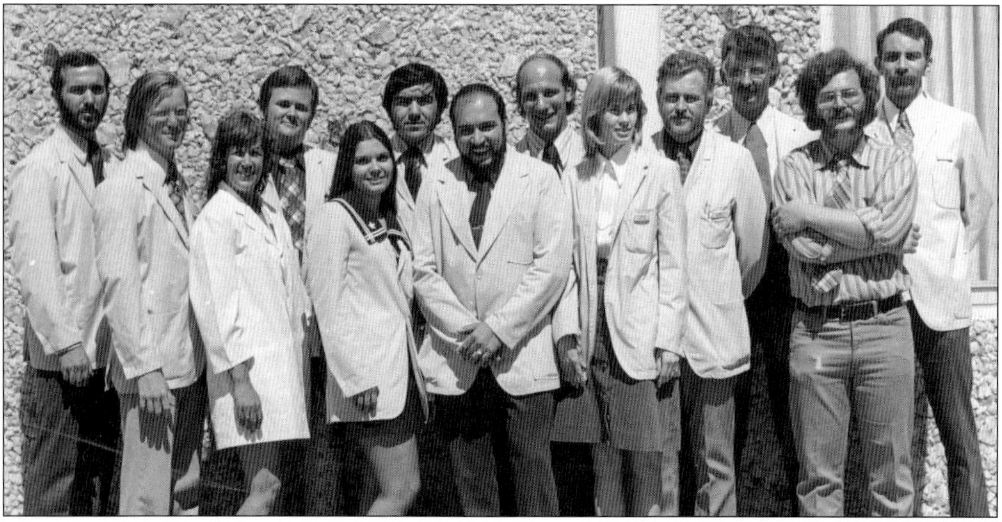

MEDEX Class 7. Through Dr. Lawrence's outreach to the School of Nursing, MEDEX accepted three experienced nurses into MEDEX Class 7. Jointly enrolled in both the MEDEX program and in the School of Nursing, these three nurses became the first students in what was to become the School of Nursing's nurse practitioner program. This photograph also shows Utah Class 1 graduate Harry Felton (second from right) as a PA faculty member.

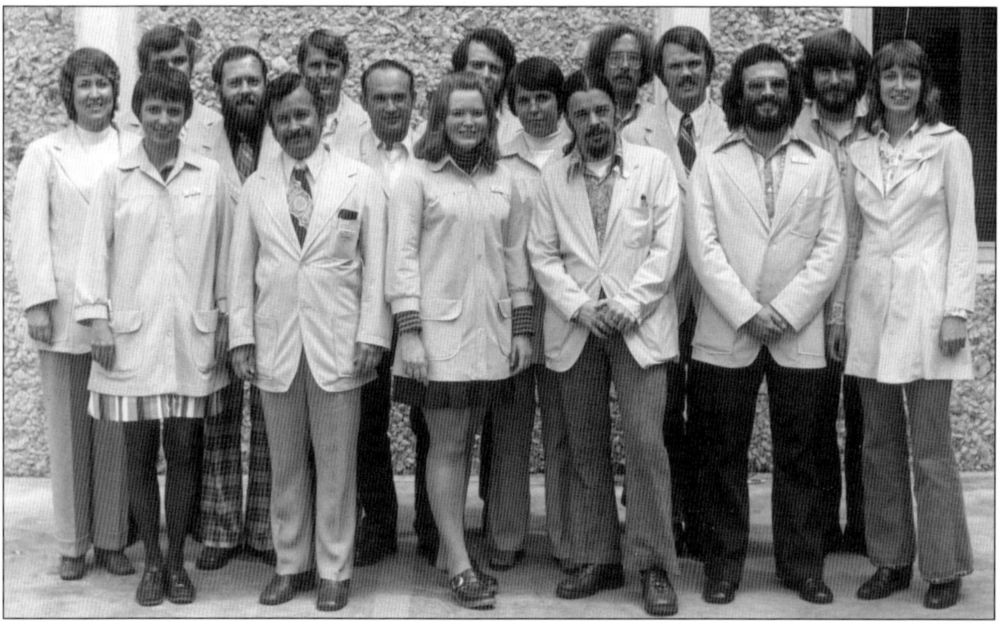

MEDEX Class 8. This photograph includes the second and final group of experienced nurses who were jointly enrolled in both MEDEX and the School of Nursing. Because of their dual training, they were eligible to practice as NPs or PAs. Also pictured is Fred "Gino" Gianola (Class 8, first row, third from right) who joined the MEDEX faculty. At far right is Barbara Coombs Lee, PA, FNP, JD, current president of Compassion and Choices.

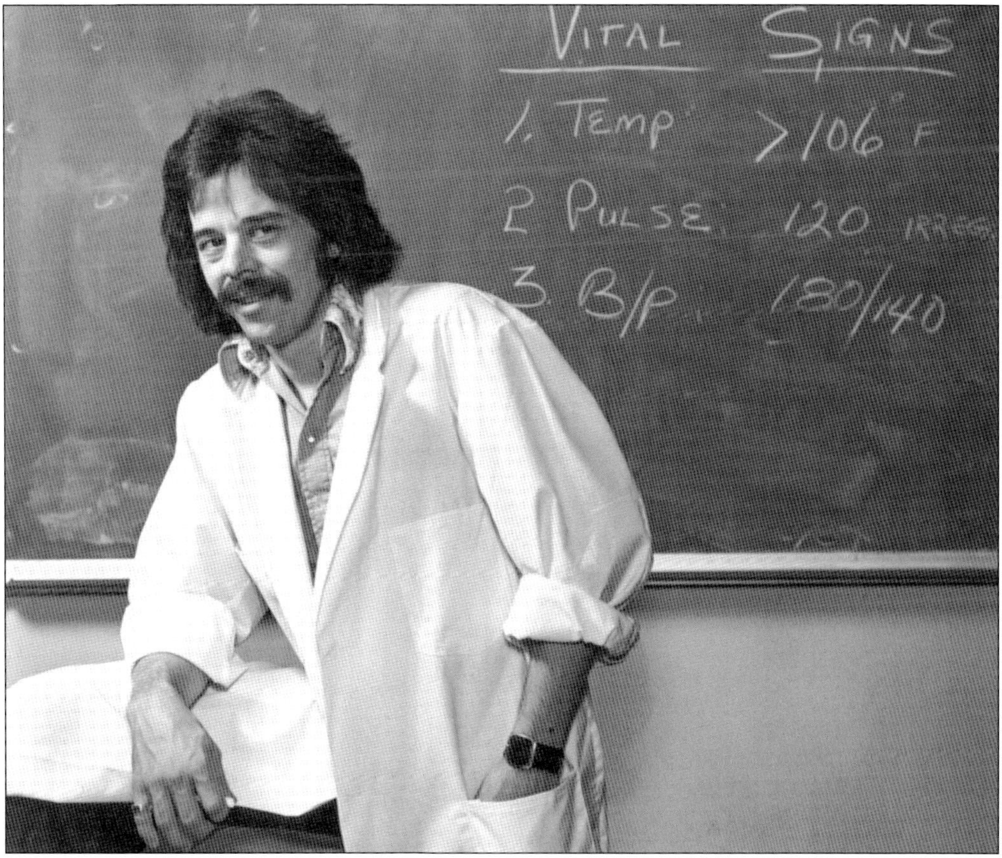
VITAL SIGNS
1. TEMP >106 F
2 PULSE 120
3. B/P 180/140

First Graduate to Join Faculty. Fred "Gino" Gianola (Class 8) is shown teaching in 1977; he still serves on the MEDEX faculty. He was the first certified PA at the National Institutes of Health and the National Cancer Institute. An active, early supporter of the Seattle Community Clinic system, he earned a master's in bioethics in 2013, and holds leadership roles for the PA History Society and the PAEA Ethics Council.

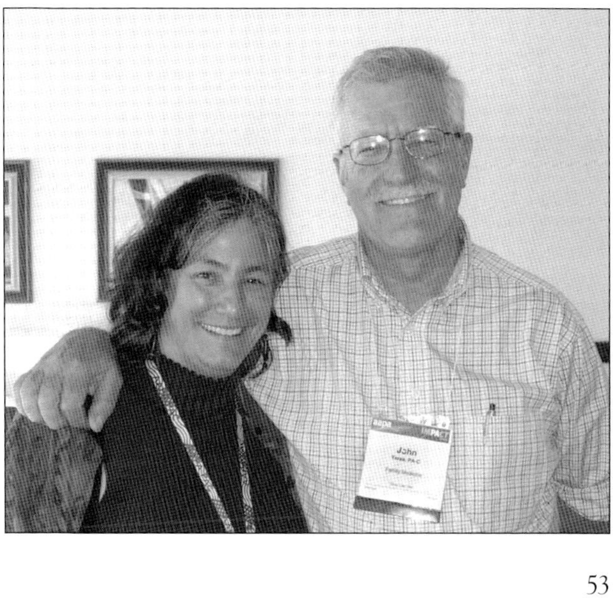

First Bachelor's Degree Recipient. In 1986, MEDEX created and received approval for its own bachelor's degree in clinical health services. The first recipient was John Yerxa (Class 18), shown here with fellow MEDEX faculty member Grace Landel. Since then, Yerxa has served as a MEDEX faculty member in Reno and in Yakima. Now living in Australia, Yerxa earned his master's degree in public health from James Cook University and has served as clinical coordinator for several primary-care medical programs.

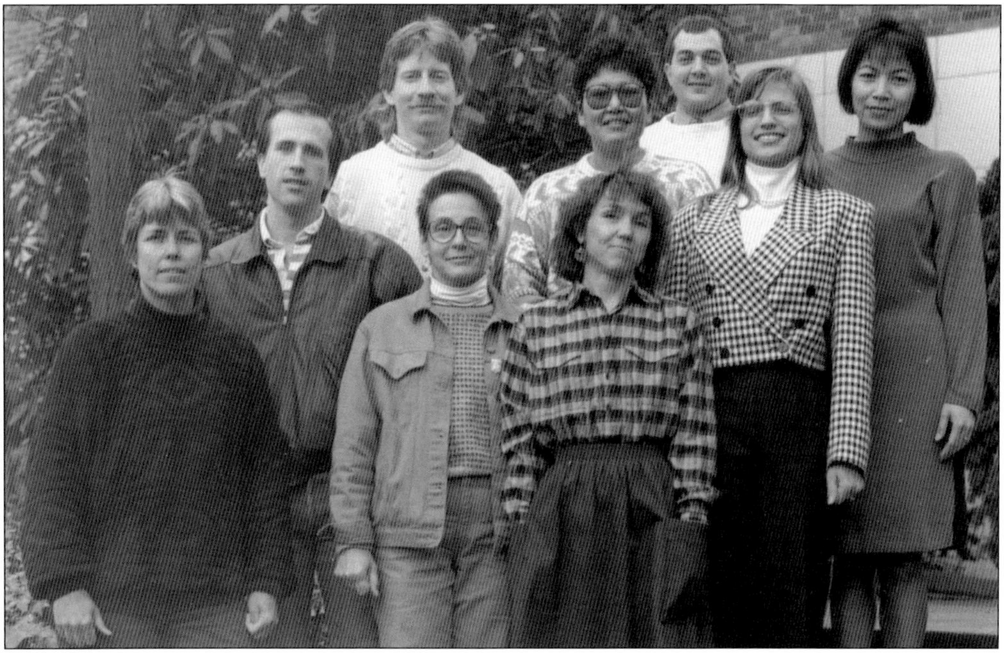

First Part-Time Class. Based on requests from applicants and employers, MEDEX created a part-time option in 1990. The part-time curriculum schedule included splitting the first year of the curriculum into 2 years (morning for the first year and afternoon for the second year), and a full-time clinical year. The first part-time class is shown here in 1993.

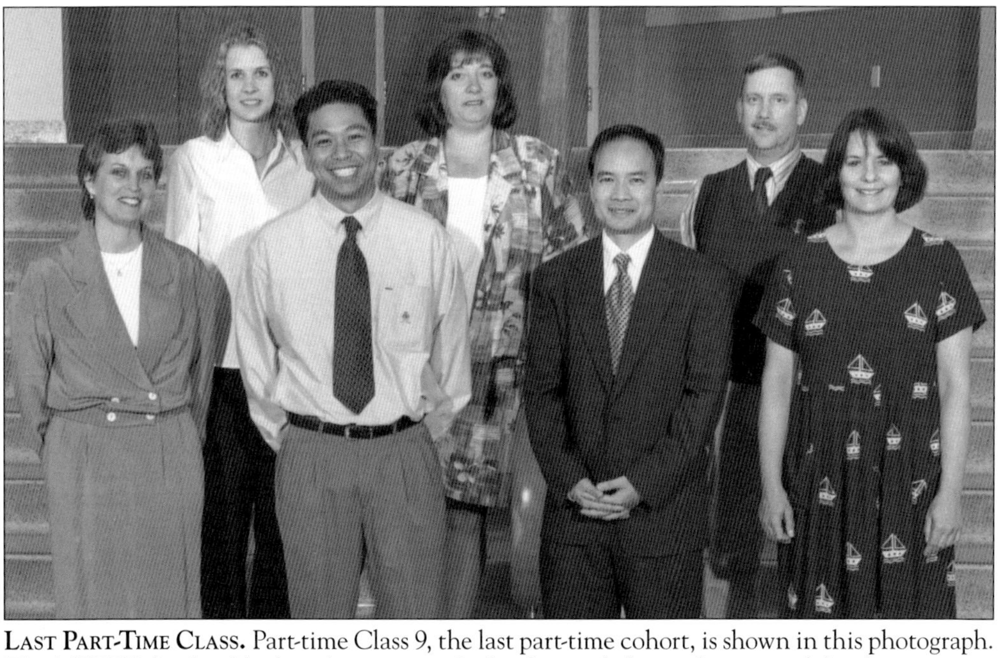

Last Part-Time Class. Part-time Class 9, the last part-time cohort, is shown in this photograph. The MEDEX faculty felt that the program had exhausted the applicant pool for the part-time option at the same time that feedback from family members indicated that the third year of full-time clinical training was difficult after students had been able to work throughout their first two years of the program.

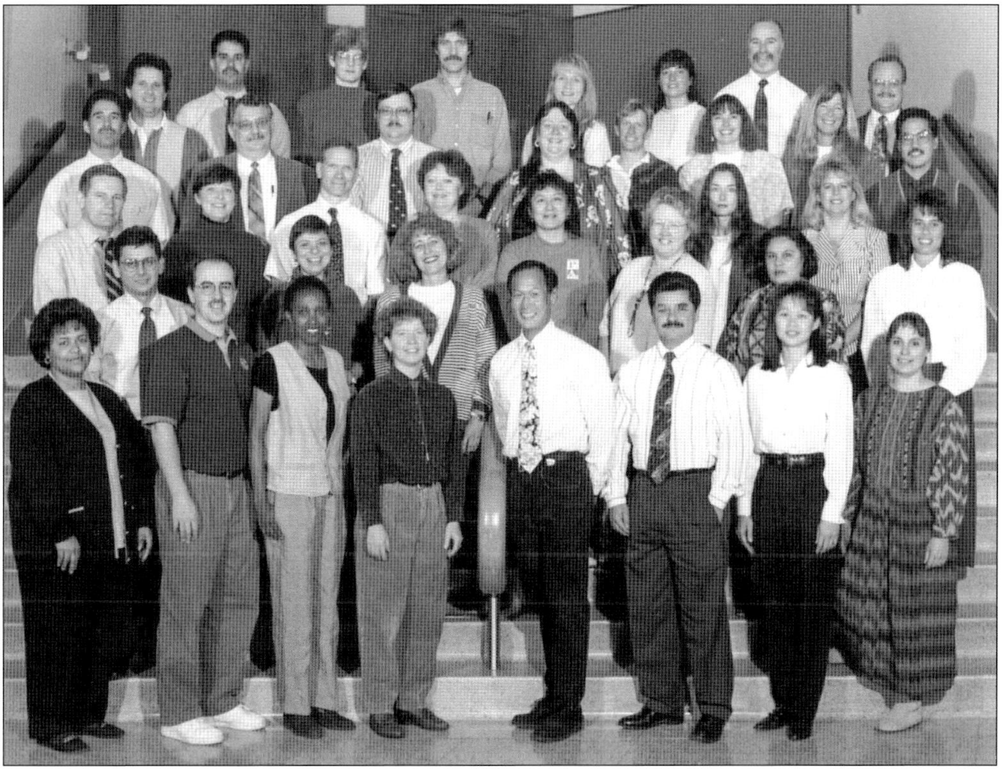

MEDEX in the School of Medicine. After more than 20 years in the School of Public Health, the changing health-care environment and new demands for a primary-care workforce brought the MEDEX program back into the School of Medicine in 1994. The program was transferred to the Department of Medical Education with dual reporting functions to the School of Medicine's dean's office. Class 28—entering in September 1994—was the first group to experience that transition.

First Spokane Master's Degrees. As more and more PA programs moved toward a master's degree as the preferred credential for PA students, MEDEX developed a new degree to be gradually phased in by the accreditation requirement of 2021. The first MEDEX master's degrees in Clinical Health Services were awarded to Seattle and Spokane students graduating in 2011. The first Spokane master's degree students, Spokane Class 13, are pictured here.

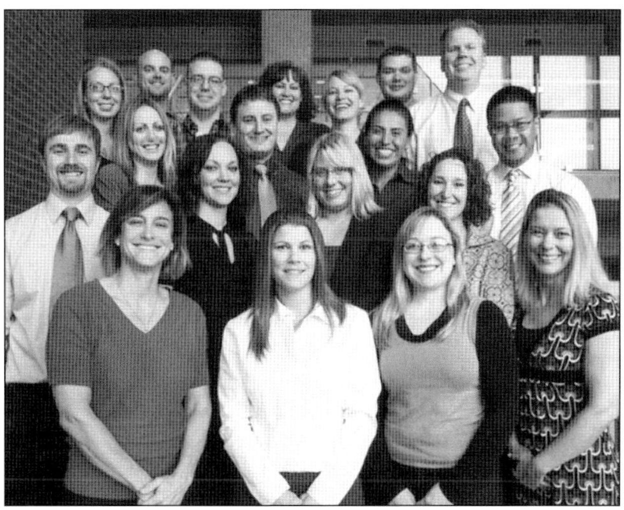

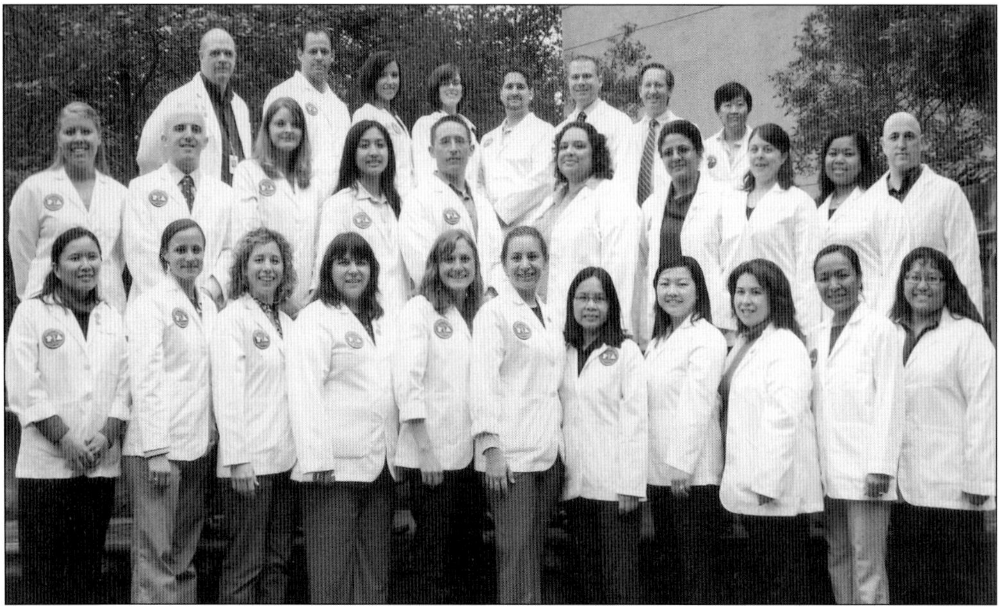

First Seattle Master's Degrees. The first Seattle MEDEX master's degree graduates, Seattle Class 43, are shown in this photograph. Beyond the bachelor's degree curriculum, master's degree students are required to complete additional coursework and writing assignments in one of four pathways: public health/prevention; rural/urban primary care; academic medicine/specialty practice; or global health.

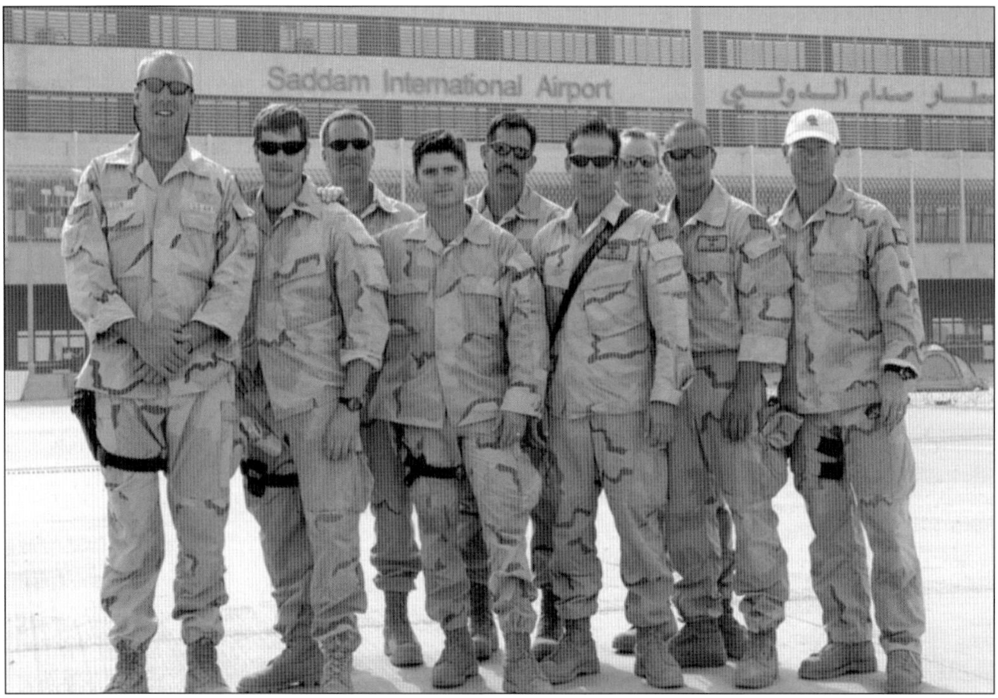

Service in Iraq. Scott Light (Class 38, fourth from left) is shown with his colleagues during Air Force deployment at Saddam (now Baghdad) International Airport. Since graduation, Light has been employed in Grays Harbor County on the Washington coast. (Courtesy of Scott Light.)

NATIONAL GUARD MEDALS. US Army veteran Alex Bertelsen served in the National Guard; during MEDEX studies, he was deployed again. Program director Ruth Ballweg (left) and administrator Jennifer Johnston (right) worked to enable him to complete requirements and graduate from MEDEX. Here, Bertelsen (center) presents National Guard medals to Ballweg and Johnston for their support. He is now a PA in orthopedics at the University of Washington Medical Center.

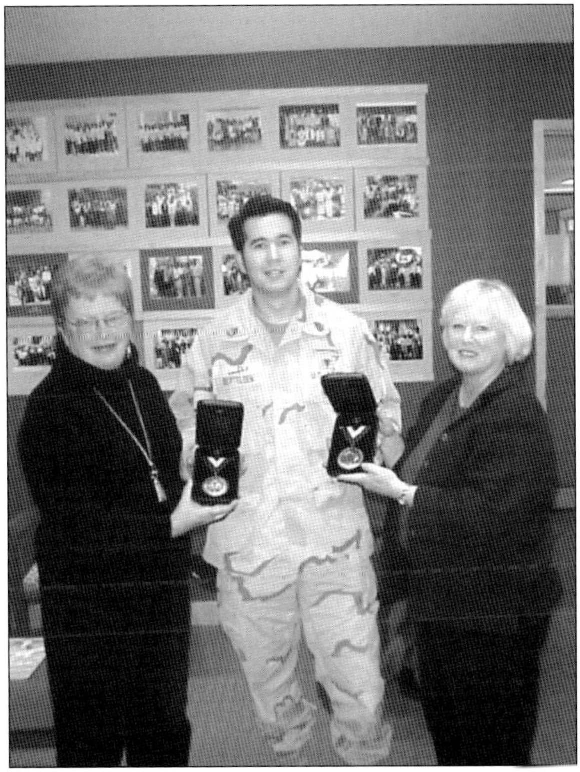

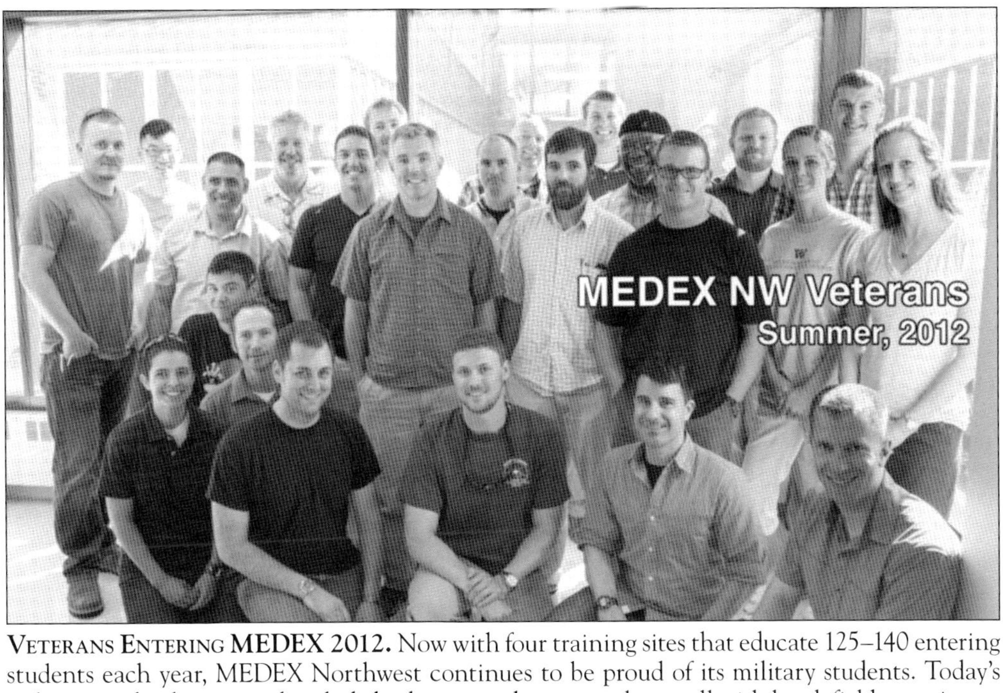

VETERANS ENTERING MEDEX 2012. Now with four training sites that educate 125–140 entering students each year, MEDEX Northwest continues to be proud of its military students. Today's military medical personnel include both men and women, almost all with battlefield experience. This photograph shows the veterans from all four Northwest Washington sites entering MEDEX in 2012 for 2014 graduation.

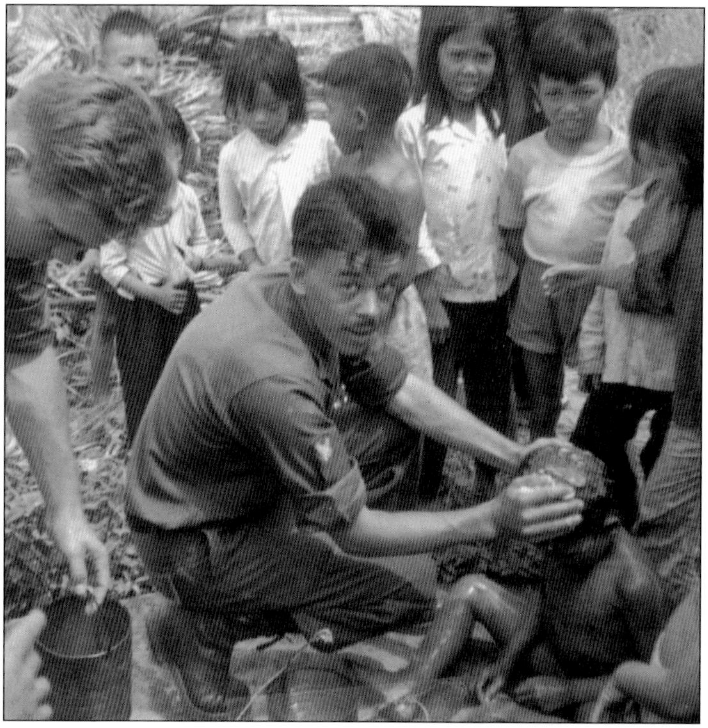

An Ounce of Prevention. Fred "Gino" Gianola cares for local children as a medical corpsman in Vietnam in 1967. He wrote to his high school suggesting that students send over "a few bars of soap." With the arrival of 2,056 bars, his off-duty clean station drew an interested crowd. He went on to work with veterans at the Seattle Veterans Administration Hospital, and is treasurer of the AAPA Veterans Caucus.

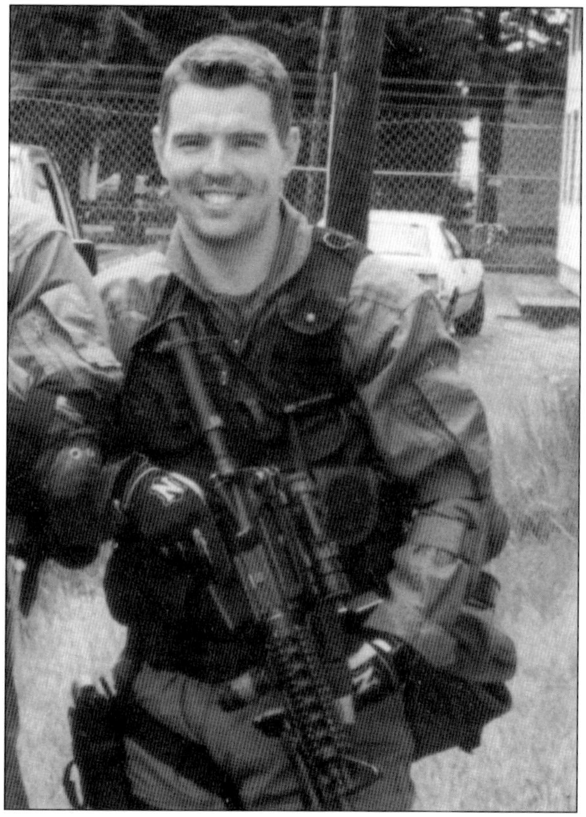

Tillman Recipient on the Faculty. Donald "D.J." Smith (Class 46) is shown at Fort Lewis in 1999. After serving as a special forces demolitions expert and special forces medic, he now works at Group Health Eastside and teaches as part-time MEDEX faculty. During MEDEX training, Smith received a Patrick Tillman Foundation scholarship. Army Ranger Patrick Tillman was an Arizona Cardinals football player who enlisted and was killed in Afghanistan.

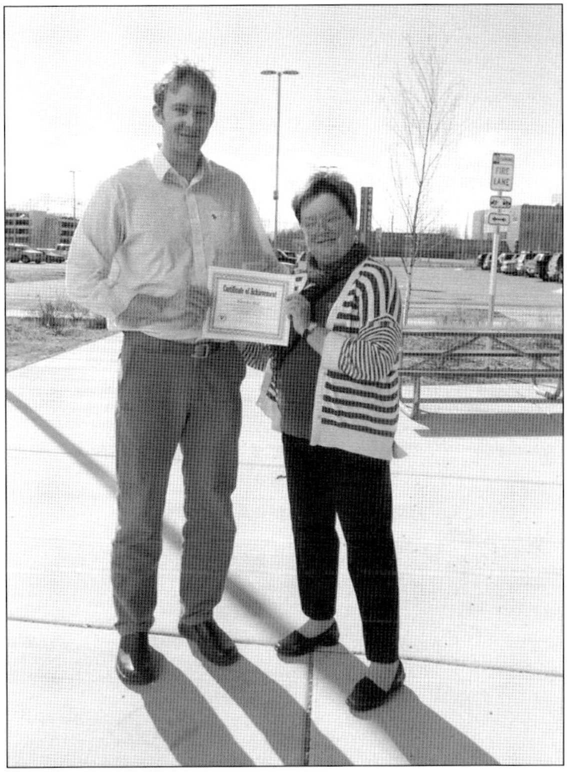

VETERAN'S CAUCUS SCHOLARSHIP RECIPIENT. Kristofer Abel (Anchorage Class 4) is presented with an AAPA Veterans Caucus at the Anchorage campus by program director Ruth Ballweg. Abel is just one of the many MEDEX graduates who have received caucus scholarships over the years from money donated by caucus members and earned from Veterans Caucus fundraisers and conferences.

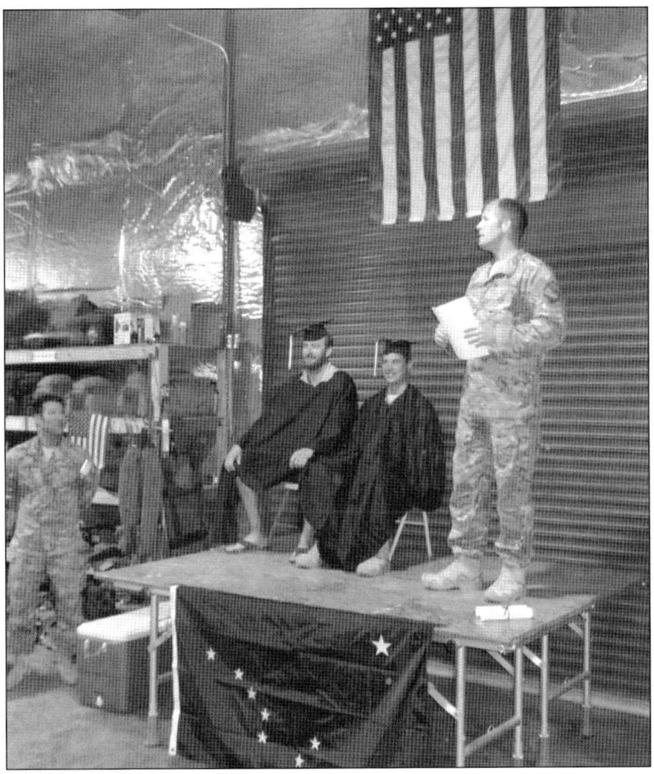

OVERSEAS GRADUATION. Two students in Anchorage Class 4 were deployed to Africa during their clinical year. MEDEX clinical coordinator Pat Hensch arranged a preceptorship in their clinic overseas, allowing both to graduate on time. On graduation day, while still deployed, they joined their Alaska cohort via Skype. Seated on stage, Kristofer Ables (left) and Nathan Greene enjoy the ceremony, arranged by colleagues on base. (Courtesy of MEDEX Alaska collection.)

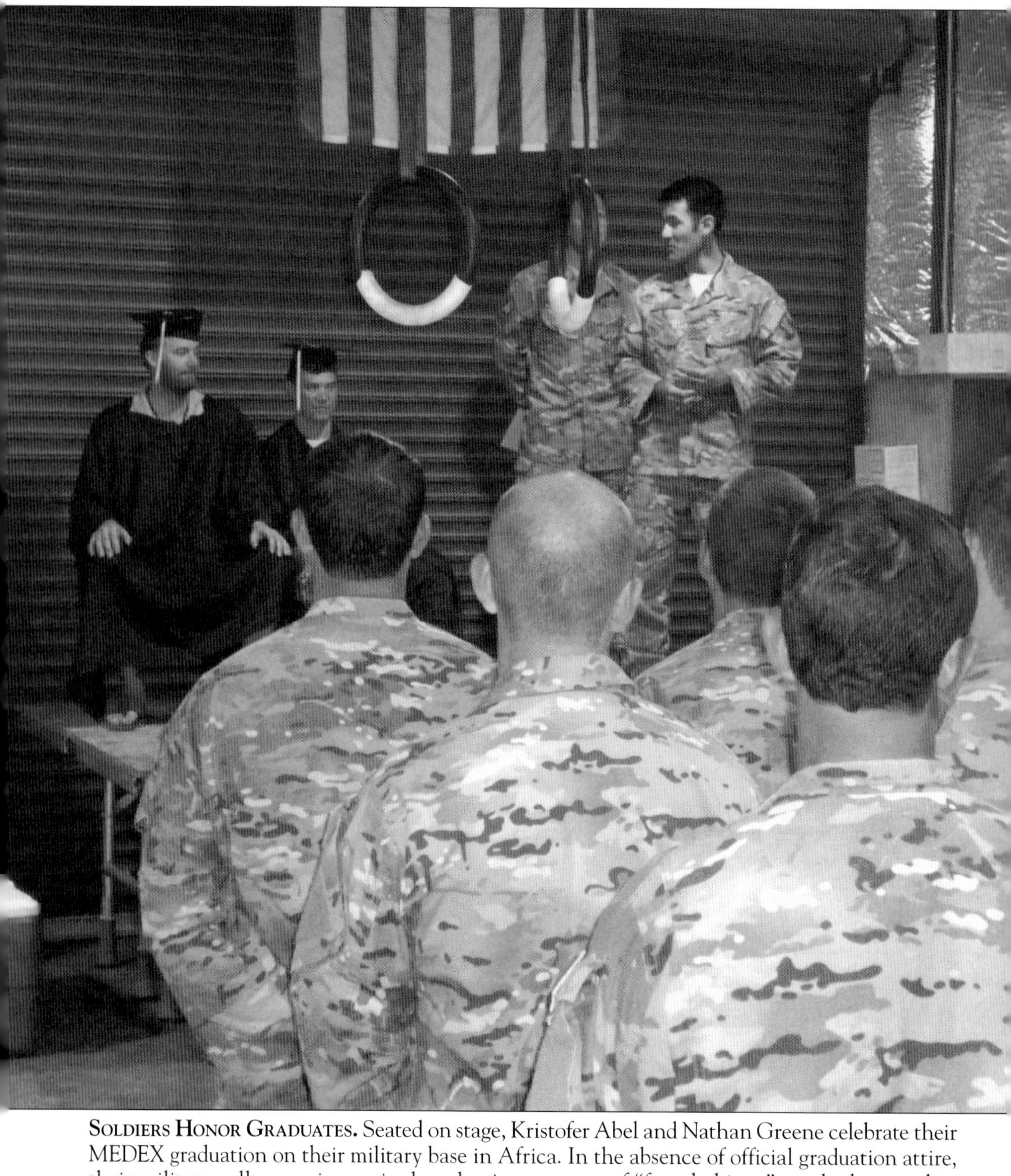

Soldiers Honor Graduates. Seated on stage, Kristofer Abel and Nathan Greene celebrate their MEDEX graduation on their military base in Africa. In the absence of official graduation attire, their military colleagues improvised graduation gear out of "found objects" on the base and in the clinic. It was a big day for everyone! (Courtesy of MEDEX Alaska collection.)

Six

Other MEDEX Projects

Dr. Richard Smith envisioned MEDEX as a nationwide network with global applications. After his work with MEDEX, he relocated to Honolulu, where he joined the faculty of the University of Hawaii with the promise that he would have the independence he sought to continue his international work. Creating MEDEX International, Dr. Smith assembled a team of global health experts—again, many of them former Peace Corps leaders—to develop and implement primary-care training programs in resource-poor countries. MEDEX International developed training materials, workshops, and a training and consultation service to expand its global networks. A range of funding was obtained including from the United States Agency for International Development (USAID) and country-specific funding to conduct needs assessments and onsite trainings. Thomas Coles (Class 1) worked with physicians and public health educators as "the first global PA." His role included training health workers in Afghanistan, Lesotho, and Guyana as well as work in Hawaii with MEDEX development activities. In the 1980s, the MEDEX Primary Care Series became the major international training tool for health workers. It was translated into 33 different languages and used in at least 84 countries.

MEDEX Northwest has continued Dr. Smith's passion and advocacy for new health workforce models. The MEDEX connection with the Alaska Community Health Practitioner Program is an extension of that commitment. In addition, MEDEX has provided consultation and guidance to over 30 US physician assistant programs on issues of primary care, diversity, and clinical training.

MEDEX's most recent workforce innovation has been a partnership with the Alaska Native Tribal Health Consortium (ANTHC) to create the first US dental therapy program. Modeled on the New Zealand program, the Alaska dental therapist program, DENTEX, is designed to train Alaska Native villagers in a two-year program to work as supervised dental extenders performing extractions, restorations, and other primary-care dental procedures. As a result of the Alaska success, the dental therapy movement is growing, despite the opposition of organized dentistry. Major health-care foundations are supporting the dental therapy movement; dental therapists are now practicing in Minnesota, and a new law was recently approved in Maine.

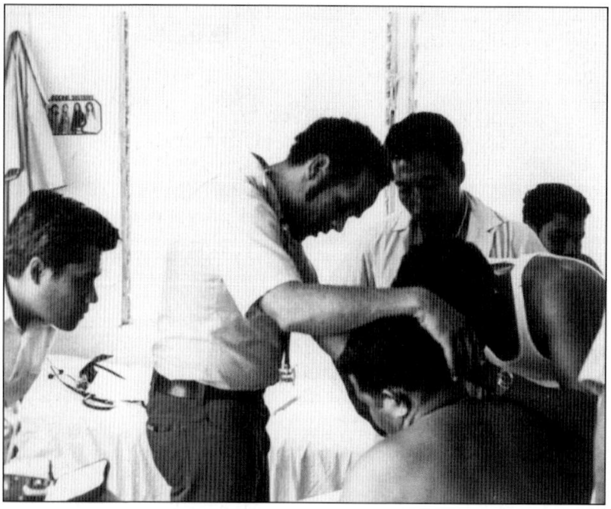

Dr. Smith in Micronesia. As a physician and public health expert, Dr. Richard Smith also spent time with the Epidemiologic Investigation Service before serving as one of the first medical directors for the Peace Corps in Africa. Here, Dr. Smith is seen in a clinical role assessing patients and serving as a teacher for local health workers. (Courtesy of the Richard Smith collection.)

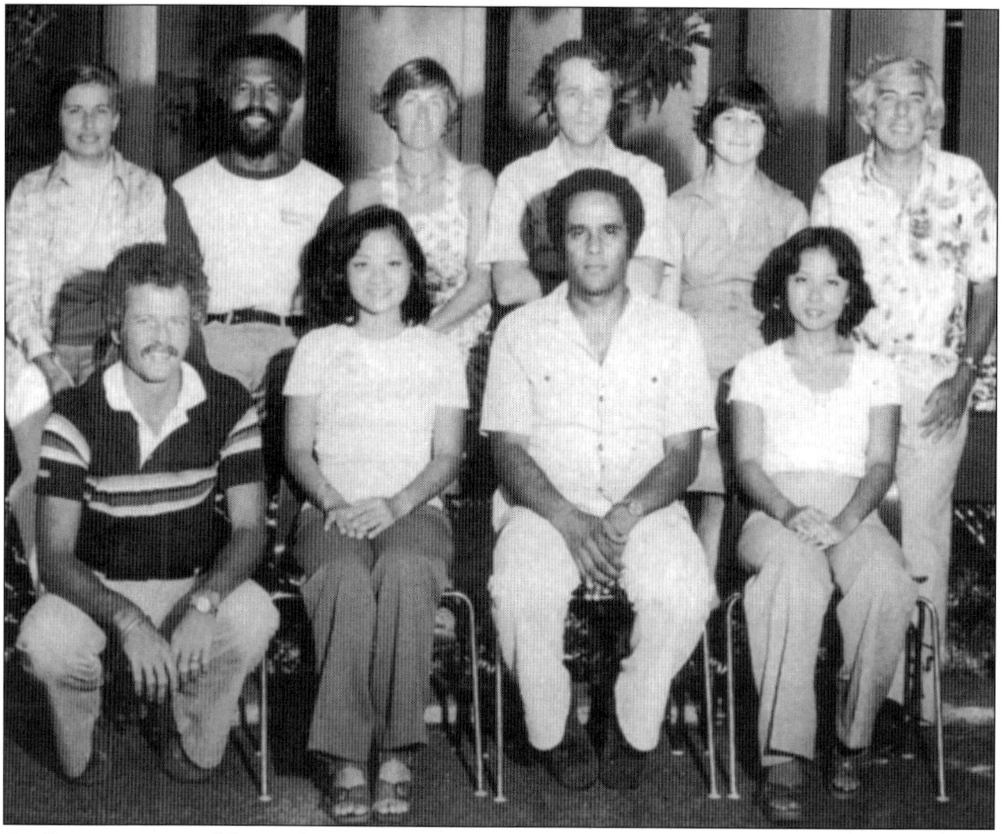

An International Vision. Leaving MEDEX Northwest with his eye on global health concerns and their solutions, Dr. Smith created MEDEX International at the University of Hawaii. Funded by the US government and a range of international sources, Dr. Smith began to create a system that included training resources for a wide range of health workers including physician assistants, nurses, and community health workers. Dr. Smith (first row, second from right) is pictured with his international team of clinicians and health educators, including Thomas Coles (first row, far left).

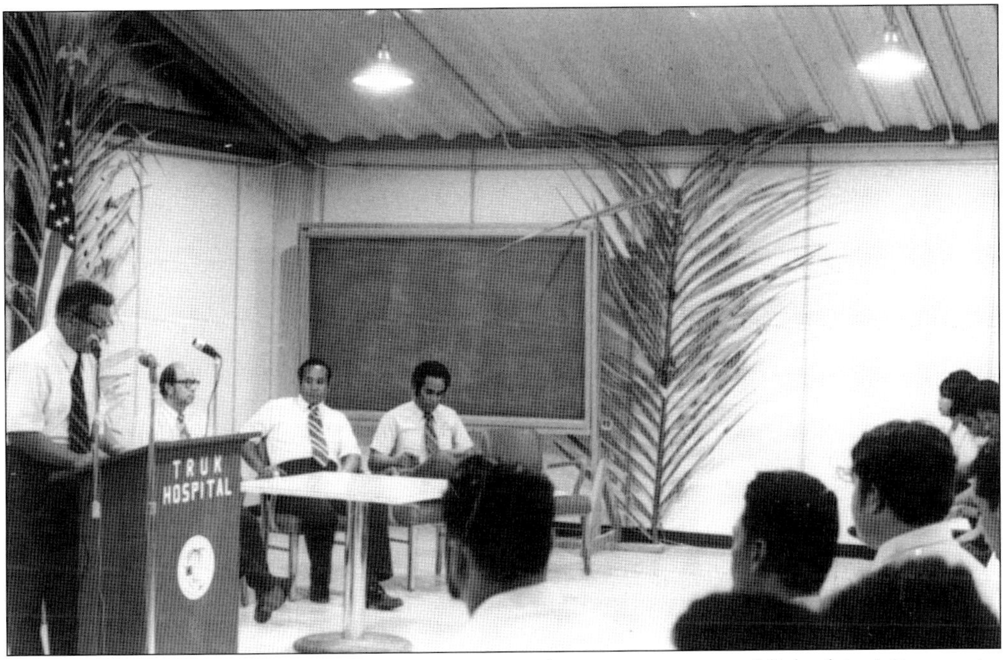

TRUK HOSPITAL. The first MEDEX international program was established in Micronesia, headquartered on the island of Truk (now Chuuk). There, the Medex practitioners were trained to support very small remote hospitals as well as clinics on the outer atolls. Here, Dr. Smith (seated at right in front of chalkboard) is in a meeting at the Truk Hospital discussing the training and utilization of the Medex.

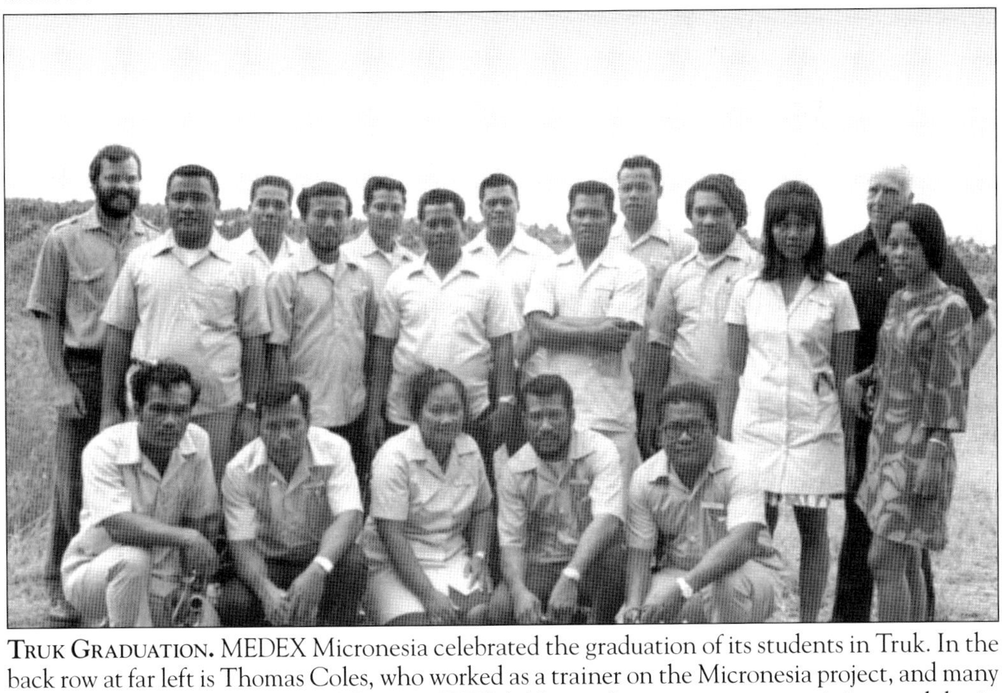

TRUK GRADUATION. MEDEX Micronesia celebrated the graduation of its students in Truk. In the back row at far left is Thomas Coles, who worked as a trainer on the Micronesia project, and many other international projects to follow. MEDEX field tested its primary care training modules in Micronesia and further expanded them to adapt to other under-resourced countries.

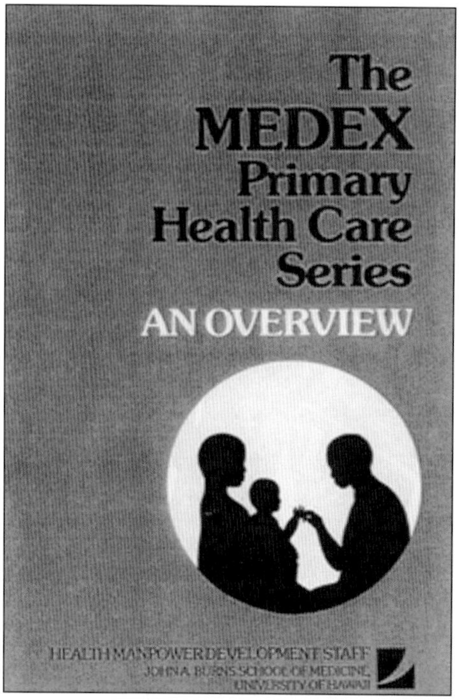

MEDEX PRIMARY CARE SERIES. The overview of the MEDEX Primary Care Series describes the use of the training materials beginning with a needs assessment and the development of a competency-based training strategy working backward from decisions about the skill set the new types of clinicians would need to learn to make a difference. Illustrations were created to maximal application in multiple countries and cultures.

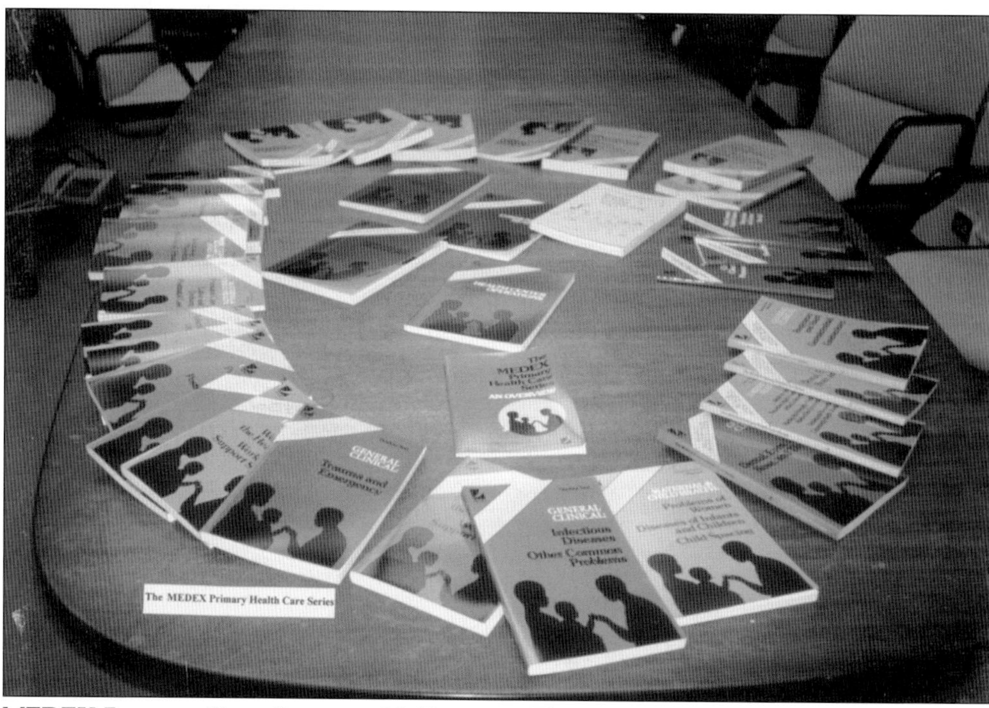

MEDEX PRIMARY CARE SERIES IN 35 VOLUMES. The MEDEX Primary Care Series is shown arrayed to demonstrate its size and complexity. Each primary-care topic was covered by separate student and trainer manuals. Ministries of health in low-resourced countries could choose the most relevant volumes, beginning with the problems most critical to their region, to prioritize their public health and primary-care delivery.

MEDEX INTERNATIONAL IN MICRONESIA. Juanito Fasong, a graduate of the MEDEX Micronesia primary health-care training program, gives a baby a well-child exam.

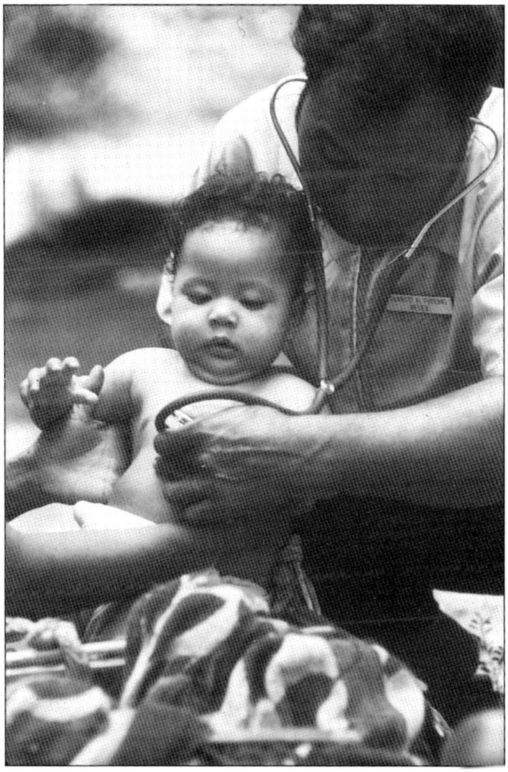

GUYANA VISITOR. In 2008, Wilton Benn, the coordinator of MEDEX and community health worker training in Guyana, visited the Department of Global Health and MEDEX. In this photograph, he is shown with MEDEX faculty members with experience with Alaska Community Health Aides Teresa Flores (Class 37) and Bill Plummer. From left to right are Teresa Flores, Ruth Ballweg, Wilton Benn, and Bill Plummer.

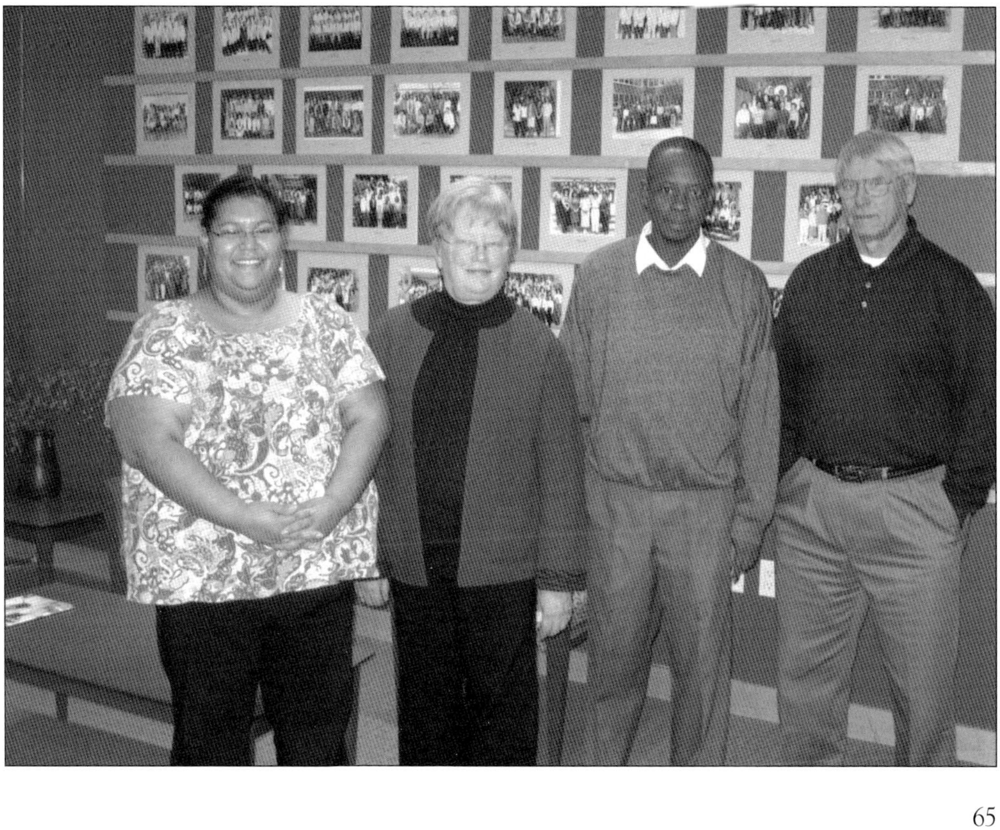

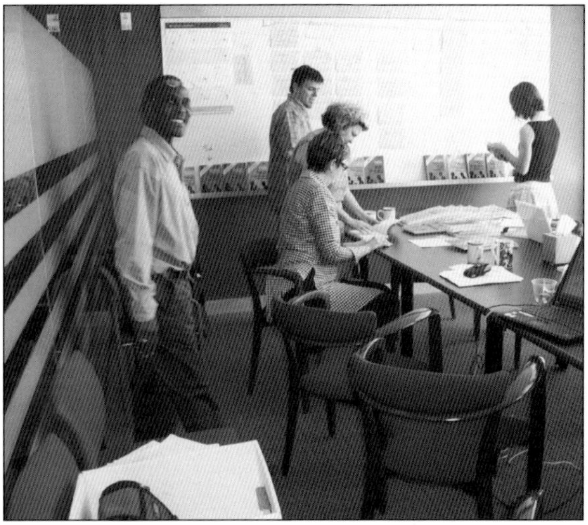

Mozambique Visitor. This MEDEX meeting, conducted in Portuguese, updated the PA/health worker training program in Mozambique. It included a representative from the Mozambique Ministry of Health (left, front); Justine Strand, head of the Duke PA program and Portuguese language consultant (seated center front); Erin Branigan, standing to the left of Strand; Chris Pupp from the Mozambique I-Tech Office with the Department of Global Health (center back near the whiteboard); and I-Tech project leader Fernanda Freistadt (right).

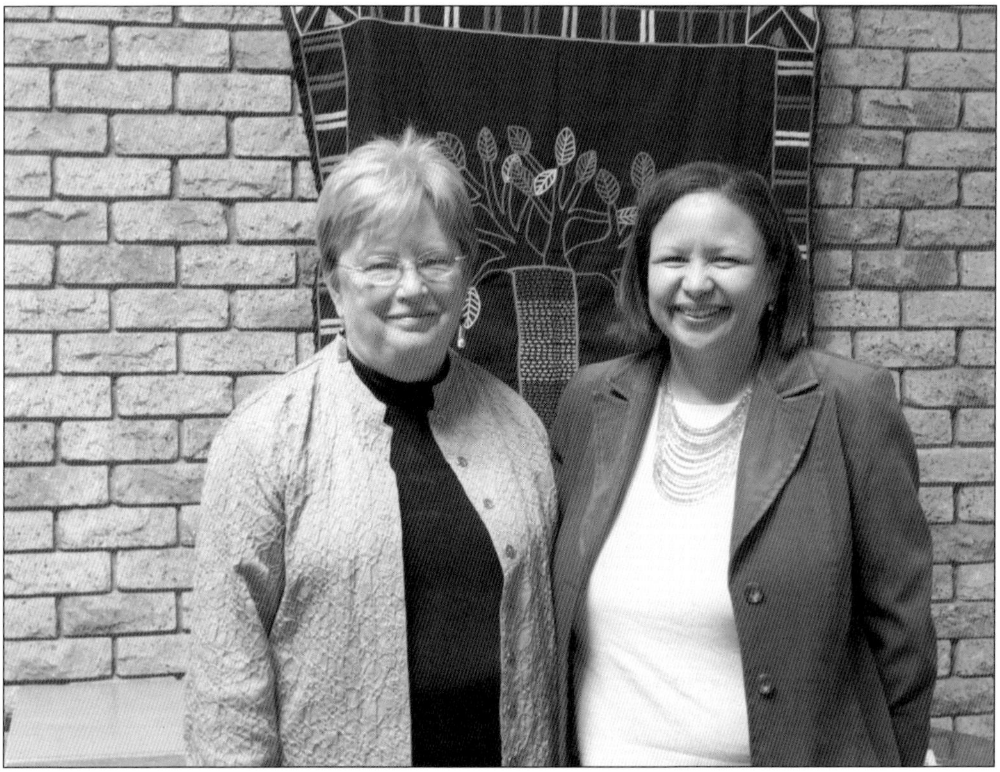

Ruth Ballweg in South Africa with Medical School Associate Dean. In 2008, Ruth Ballweg was plenary speaker for the first Conference on Clinical Associates in Johannesburg, celebrating three new PA programs at the University of Pretoria, the University of Witwatersrand, and Charles Sisulu University. She also lectured at the University of Capetown and met with the International Medical Regulatory Agencies (IAMRA). Here, she meets with Dr. Gonda Perez, deputy dean of the University of Capetown School of Medicine. (Author's collection.)

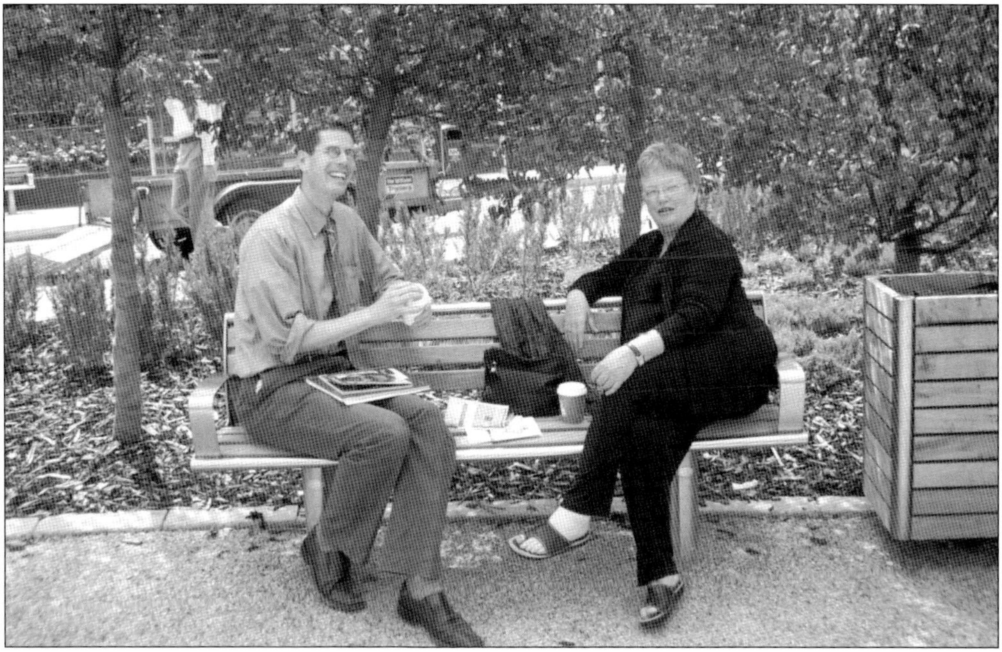

St. George's Hospital, United Kingdom. MEDEX connected with developing programs in the United Kingdom to provide support and encouragement. Joel Grey, the founding director of the St. George's PA program in London, is seen in the hospital courtyard with Ruth Ballweg. St. George's was the only PA-led program in all the British programs.

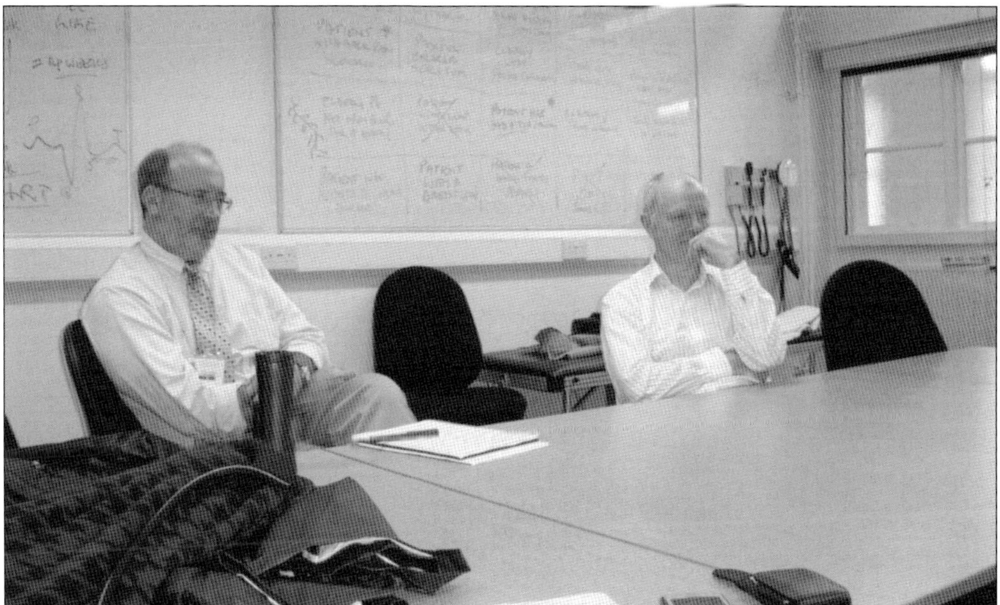

Birmingham Program. The University of Birmingham School of Medicine developed another of the first PA programs in Britain under the leadership of Dr. James Parle and medical education leader Nick Ross. US physician assistant David Kuhns soon joined them as a faculty member and PA role model. Kuhns is seen here on the left with Dr. Parle. Birmingham worked closely with a neighboring PA program at Wolverhampton University led by Phil Begg. (Author's collection.)

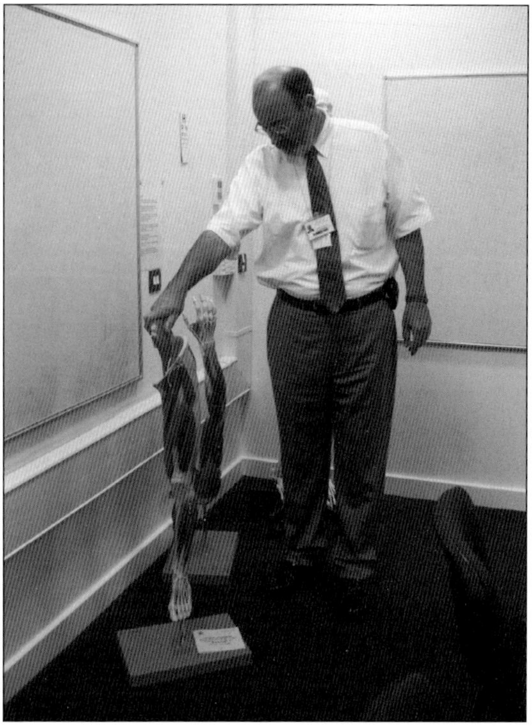

Kuhns in Birmingham. David Kuhns, MPH, PA-C, has been active in the development of PA educational programs in the United Kingdom. Kuhns has also been a part of the MEDEX global health pathway, where he served as a lecturer and capstone advisor. A graduate of the St. Louis PA program, Kuhns is now the director of the new PA program at the Royal College of Surgeons in Dublin, Ireland. (Author's collection.)

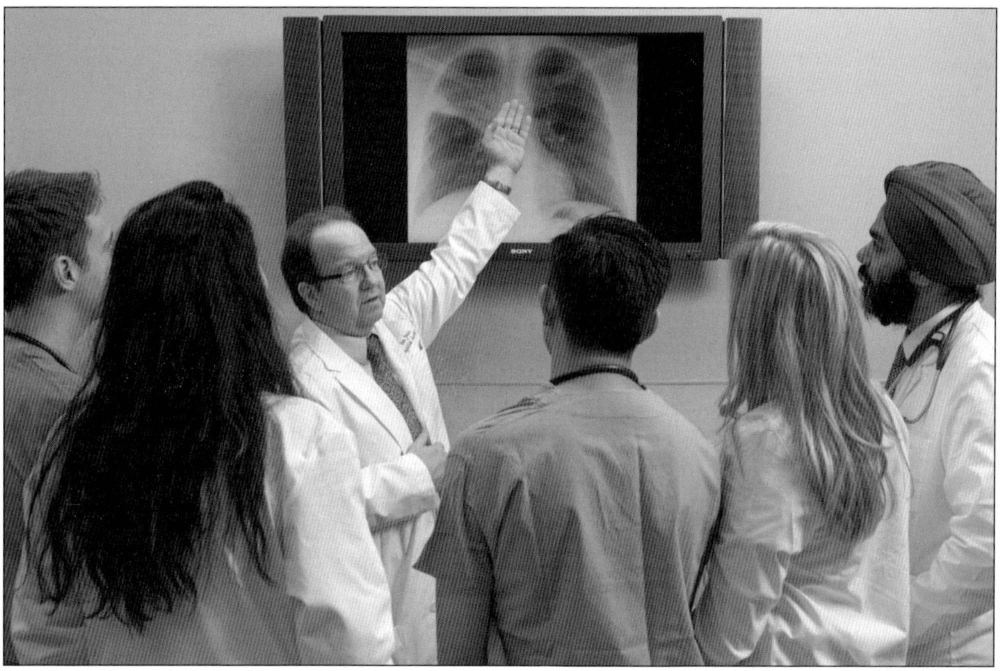

Winnipeg Program. Ian Jones (Class 30) teaches as director of the University of Manitoba PA program in Winnipeg, which opened in 2004. Jones served as first civilian president of the Canadian Academy of Physician Assistants; prior officers were graduates of the Canadian Forces PA program. In 2014, Alberta passed legislation for PA practice. Ontario has programs at McMaster University and the University of Toronto. (Courtesy of Ian Jones.)

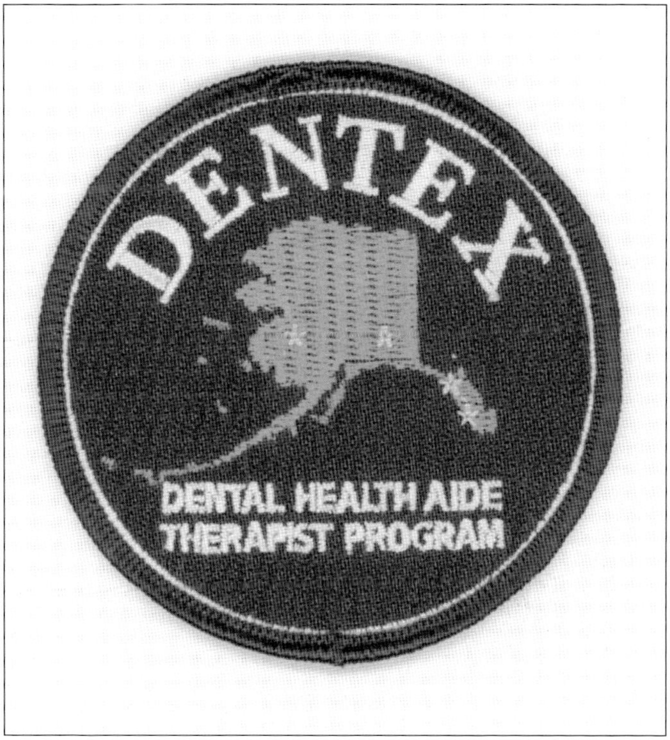

DENTEX Logo. While not previously known in the United States, the dental therapy career was introduced to Alaska in 2004 through an agreement with the University of Otago in New Zealand. The Alaska Native Tribal Health Consortium (ANTHC) sent two cohorts of Alaska trainees to New Zealand. After their two-year program, these dental health aide therapists (DHATs) returned to Alaska to practice. MEDEX Northwest partnered with the ANTHC to create a dental therapy program in Alaska to serve Alaska Native communities. (Courtesy of the DENTEX collection.)

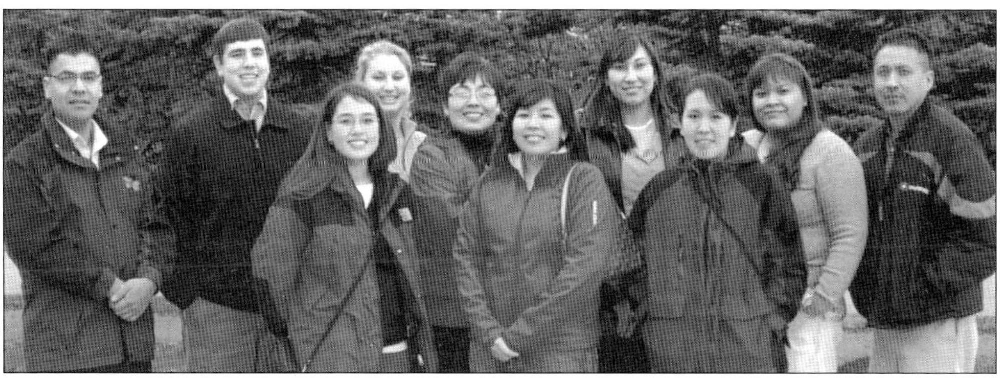

New Zealand Dental Therapy Students. These Alaska students were trained as dental therapists in New Zealand. From left to right are Brian James, Conan Murat, Kimberly Baldwin, Stephanie Woods, Aurora Johnson, Tammy Gologergen, Rochelle Ferry, Alicia Active, Lillian McGilton, and Bobby Curtis. (Courtesy of the DENTEX collection.)

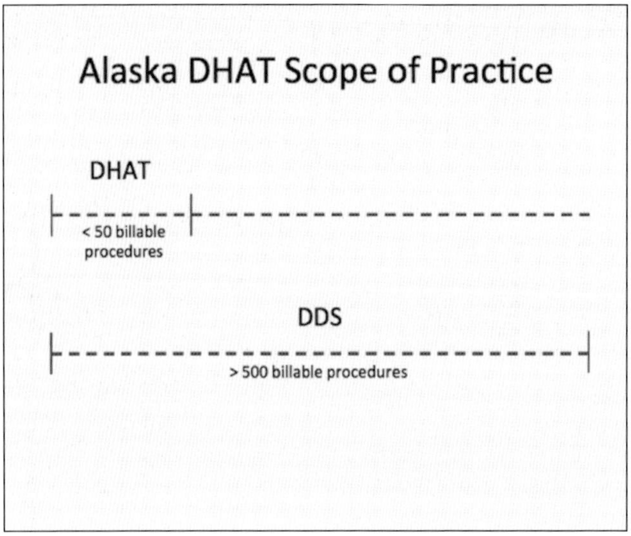

DHAT/Dentist Comparison. With a relatively short two-year training period, the scope of practice for DENTEX or DHATs is only a small portion of a dentist's large skill set. This illustration compares the scope of practice for the two roles. A key requirement of dental therapy practice is supervised practice by a licensed dentist. In remote Alaska villages, that supervision may be carried out using telemedicine equipment connecting the therapist to a dentist in a regional center. (Courtesy of the DENTEX collection.)

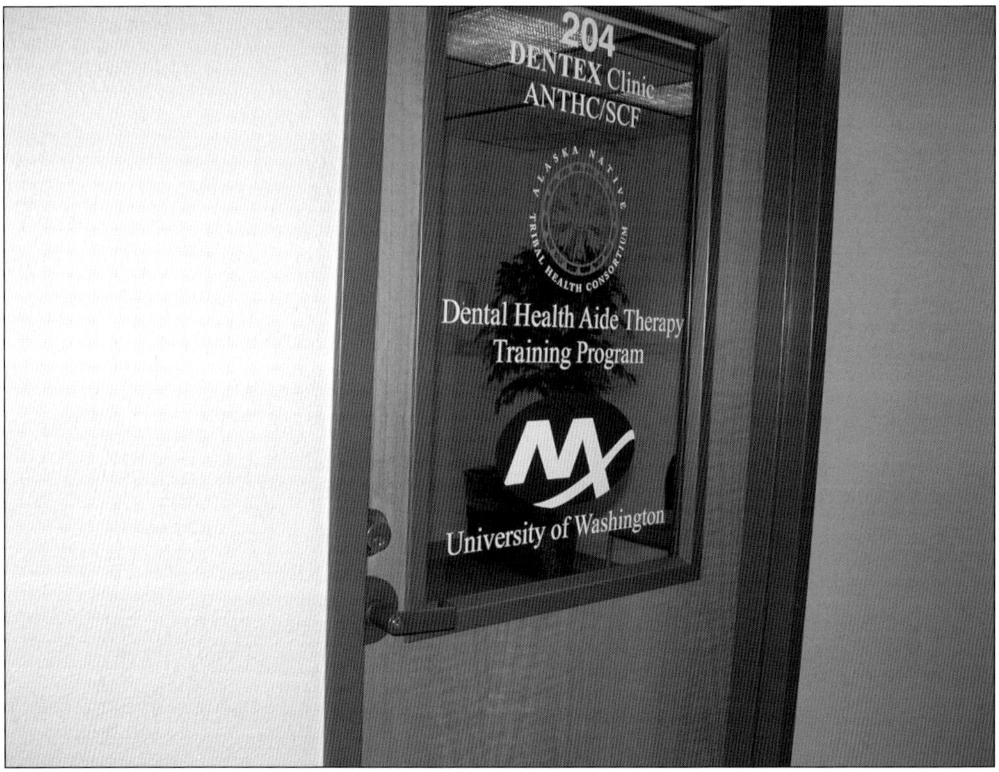

DENTEX Clinic Door. The education of Alaska DHATs is split between one year in Anchorage and one year in Bethel, Alaska. Students then complete a four-month full-time clinical preceptorship with a dentist in a third setting. Pictured is the door to the Alaska DENTEX clinic, classroom, and offices. The signage clearly designates the partnership of the Alaska Native Tribal Health Consortium (ANTHC) and the MEDEX program at the University of Washington. (Courtesy of the DENTEX collection.)

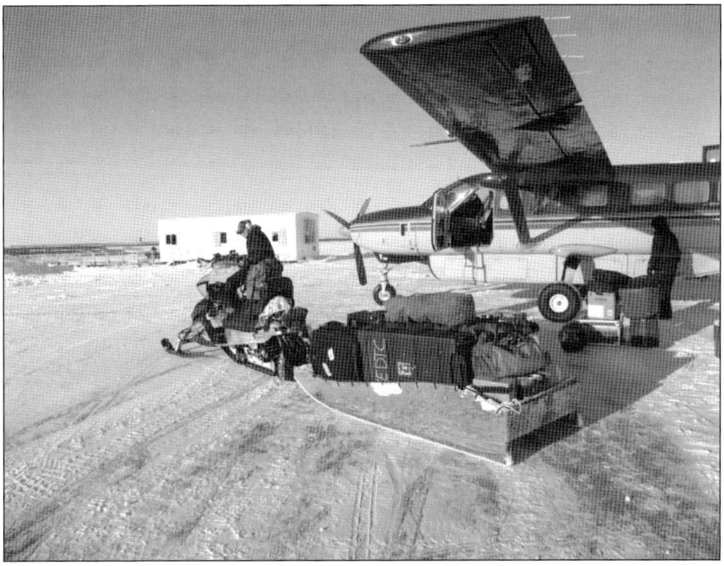

Care for All Seasons. A DENTEX sled arrives at a landing field ready for use and packed with supplies for a traveling dental clinic. Students bring their own supplies for clinical rotations as training for their careers in mobile dentistry services, bringing care where it is most needed on all roads and no roads at all. (Courtesy DENTEX collection.)

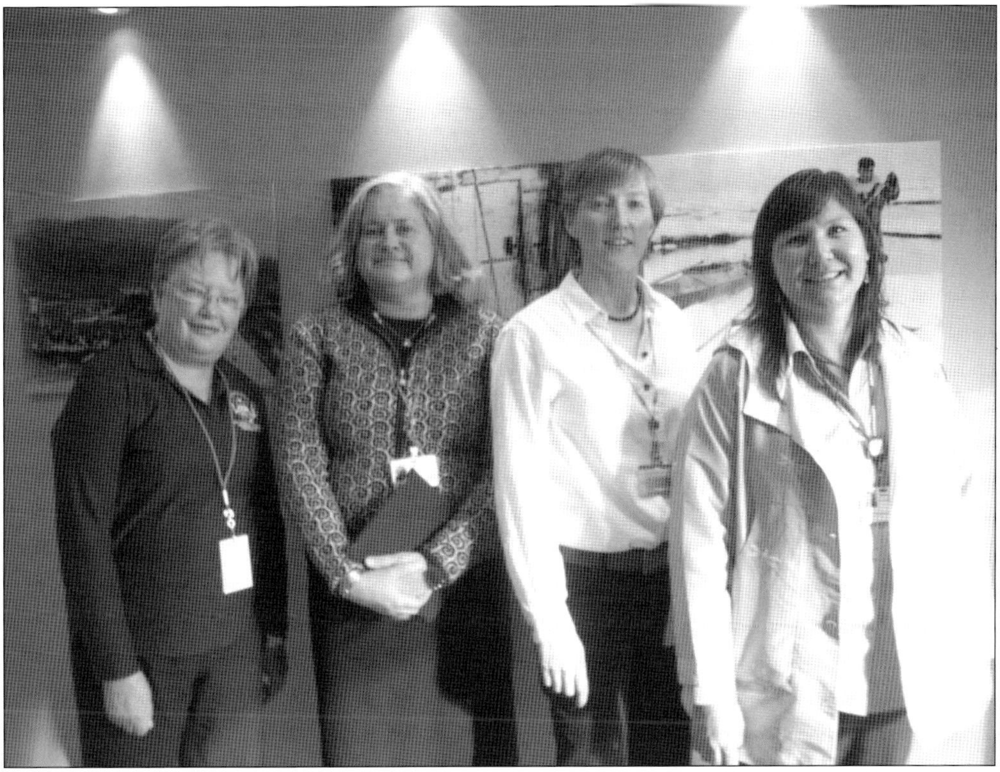

Alaska Collaboration. The creation of DENTEX involved the collaboration of leaders from ANTHC and from MEDEX. One key player was MEDEX administrator Jennifer Johnston, who is not shown in this photograph. Others included are, from left to right, MEDEX director Ruth Ballweg; the leader of the ANTHC Health Aide program, Victoria Hart; Dr. Mary Williard, public health dentist; and Val Davidson, then senior director of intergovernmental and legal affairs for ANTHC (presently commissioner for the Alaska Department of Health and Social Services). (Author's collection.)

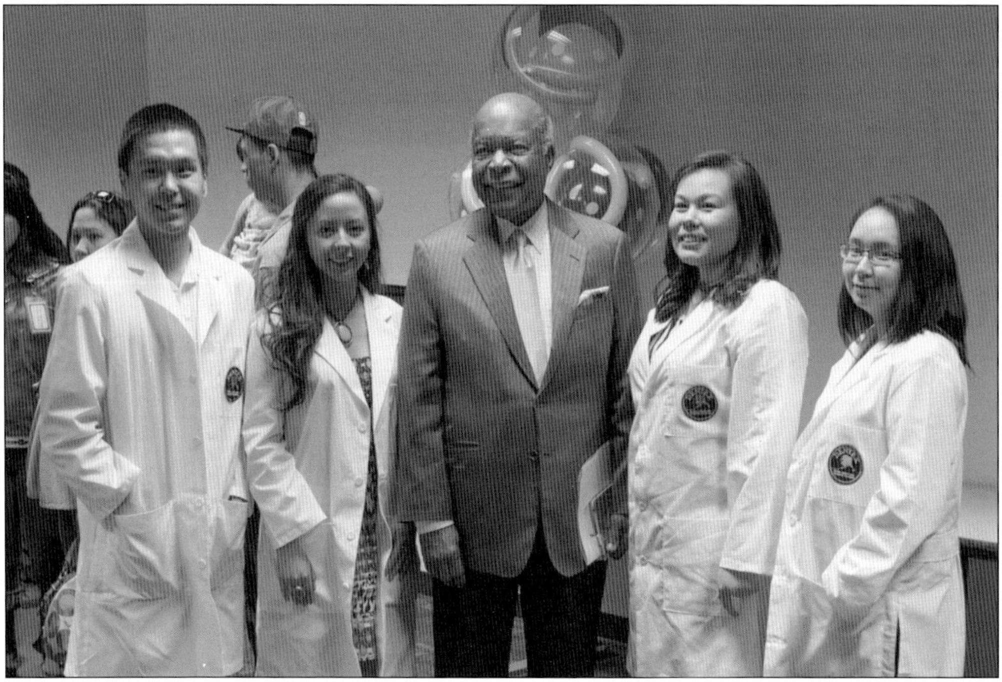

Dr. Sullivan at DENTEX. Dr. Louis Sullivan, the former secretary of the federal government's Department of Health and Human Services, along with many other national public health leaders, served as an important advocate for the dental therapy program. Dr. Sullivan gave the keynote address for the 10th anniversary event at ANTHC headquarters in Anchorage and is pictured with, from left to right, Charles Redfox, Sabrina Chilton, Sadie Green, and Carrie Tikiun. (Courtesy of the DENTEX collection.)

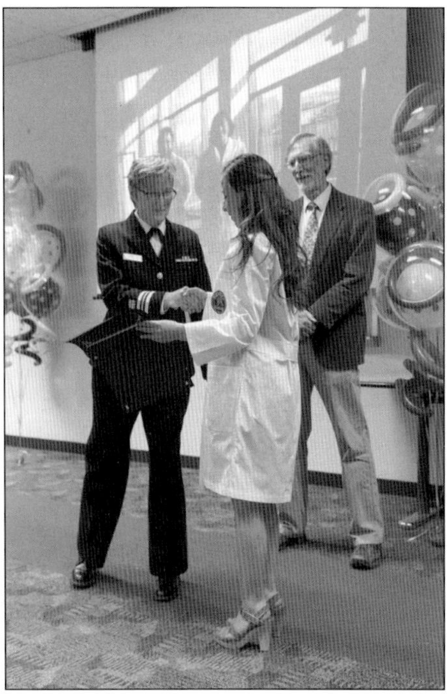

DENTEX Anniversary. The 10th anniversary celebration also featured the graduation of the newest DENTEX class. In this photograph, Dr. Mary Williard is seen presenting the graduation certificate to Sabrina Chilton with Dr. Louis Fiset in the background. (Courtesy of the DENTEX collection.)

DENTEX White Coat Ceremony. Dr. Louis Fiset, the DENTEX curriculum developer, works for MEDEX in Seattle but spends time with the DENTEX students during both their first and second years. In addition to creating the curriculum—based on the New Zealand dental therapy model—Dr. Fiset also evaluates the students in their clinical training and provides assistance with their community-based research and writing assignments. The occasion is the transition ceremony, the presentation of "official white coats" to students who have completed the first year and are moving on to the clinical year. (Courtesy of the DENTEX collection.)

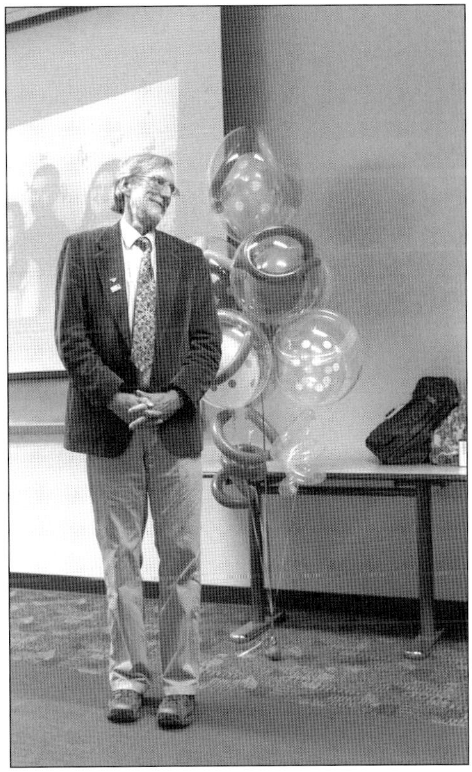

Moose in Anchorage. Alaska Native students from remote villages always enjoy seeing the moose that wander through urban Anchorage in the winter. Two adult moose are seen here outside student apartments near the University of Alaska campus. (Courtesy of the DENTEX collection.)

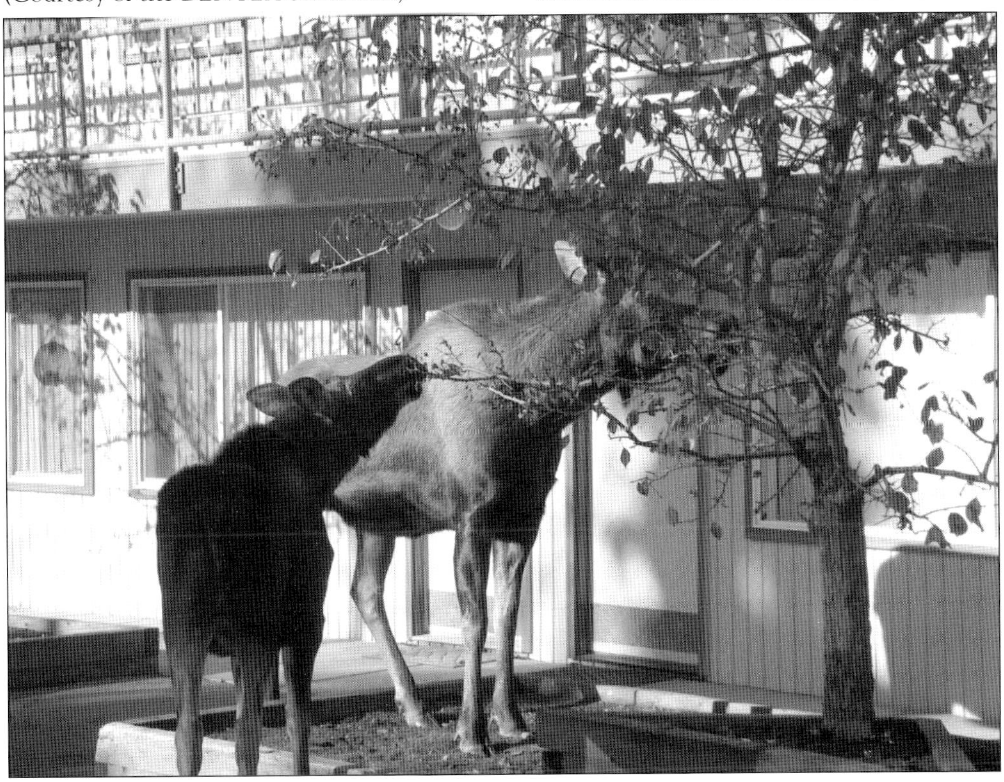

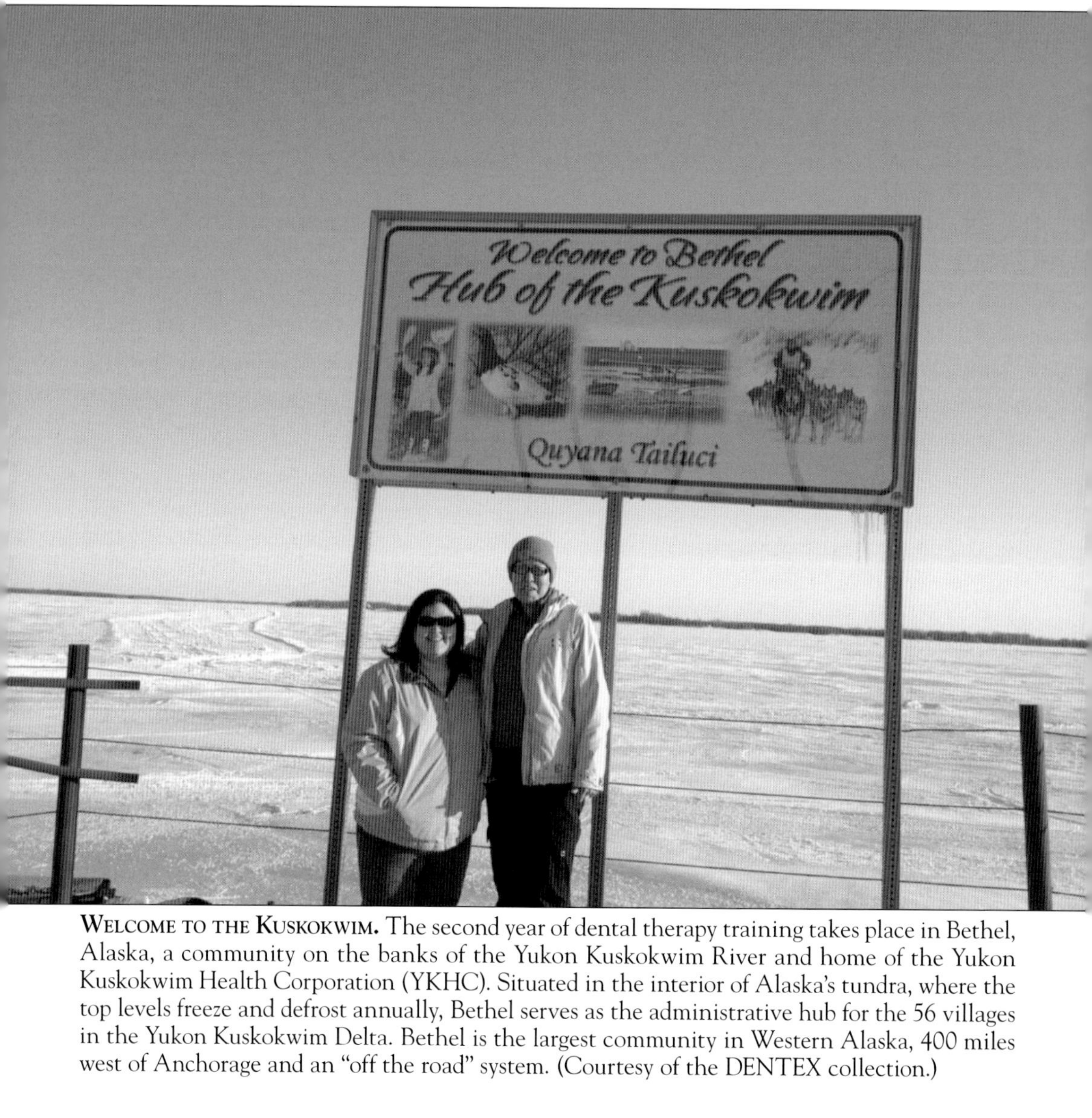

Welcome to the Kuskokwim. The second year of dental therapy training takes place in Bethel, Alaska, a community on the banks of the Yukon Kuskokwim River and home of the Yukon Kuskokwim Health Corporation (YKHC). Situated in the interior of Alaska's tundra, where the top levels freeze and defrost annually, Bethel serves as the administrative hub for the 56 villages in the Yukon Kuskokwim Delta. Bethel is the largest community in Western Alaska, 400 miles west of Anchorage and an "off the road" system. (Courtesy of the DENTEX collection.)

Dr. Shoffstall-Cone. US Public Health Service doctor Sarah Shoffstall-Cone, DDS, MPH, is the DENTEX clinical site director and splits her time between Anchorage and Bethel. She is pictured presenting at the 10th anniversary of the DHAT program in Anchorage in June 2014. (Courtesy of the DENTEX collection.)

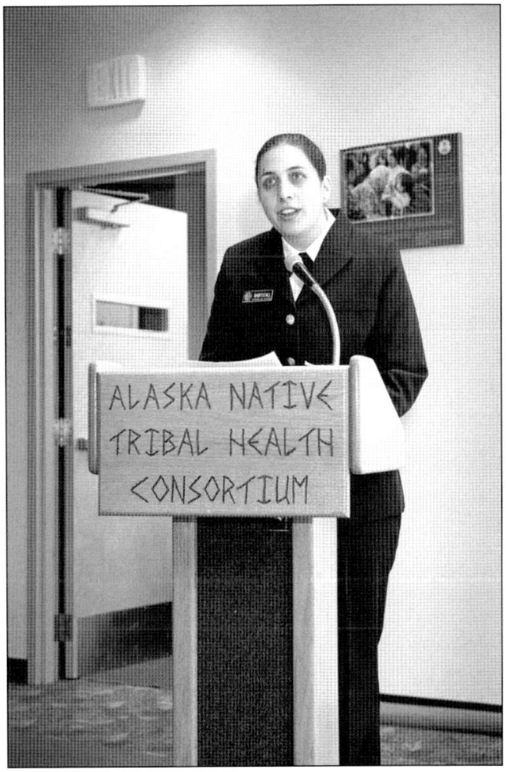

Student with Dental Model. Dental training includes extensive work with sculptured dental models before the student moves on to working with real patients. In the meantime, students learn dental examinations on live patients with supervision. Here, a DENTEX student is shown working on a dental model to practice procedures and positioning. (Courtesy of the DENTEX collection.)

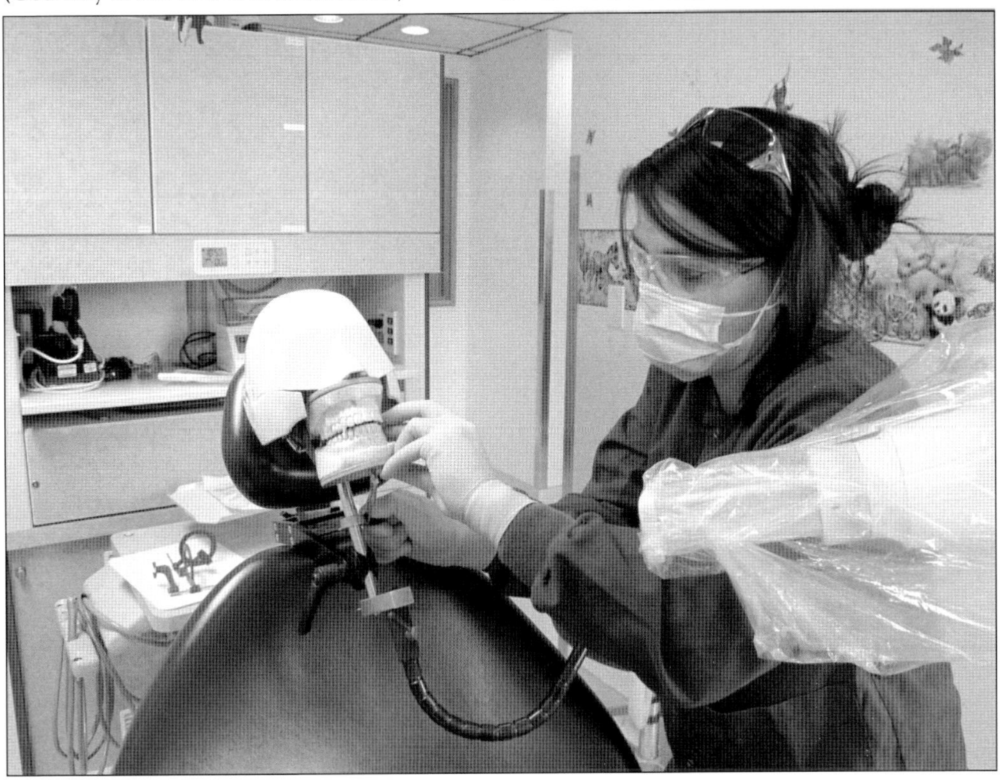

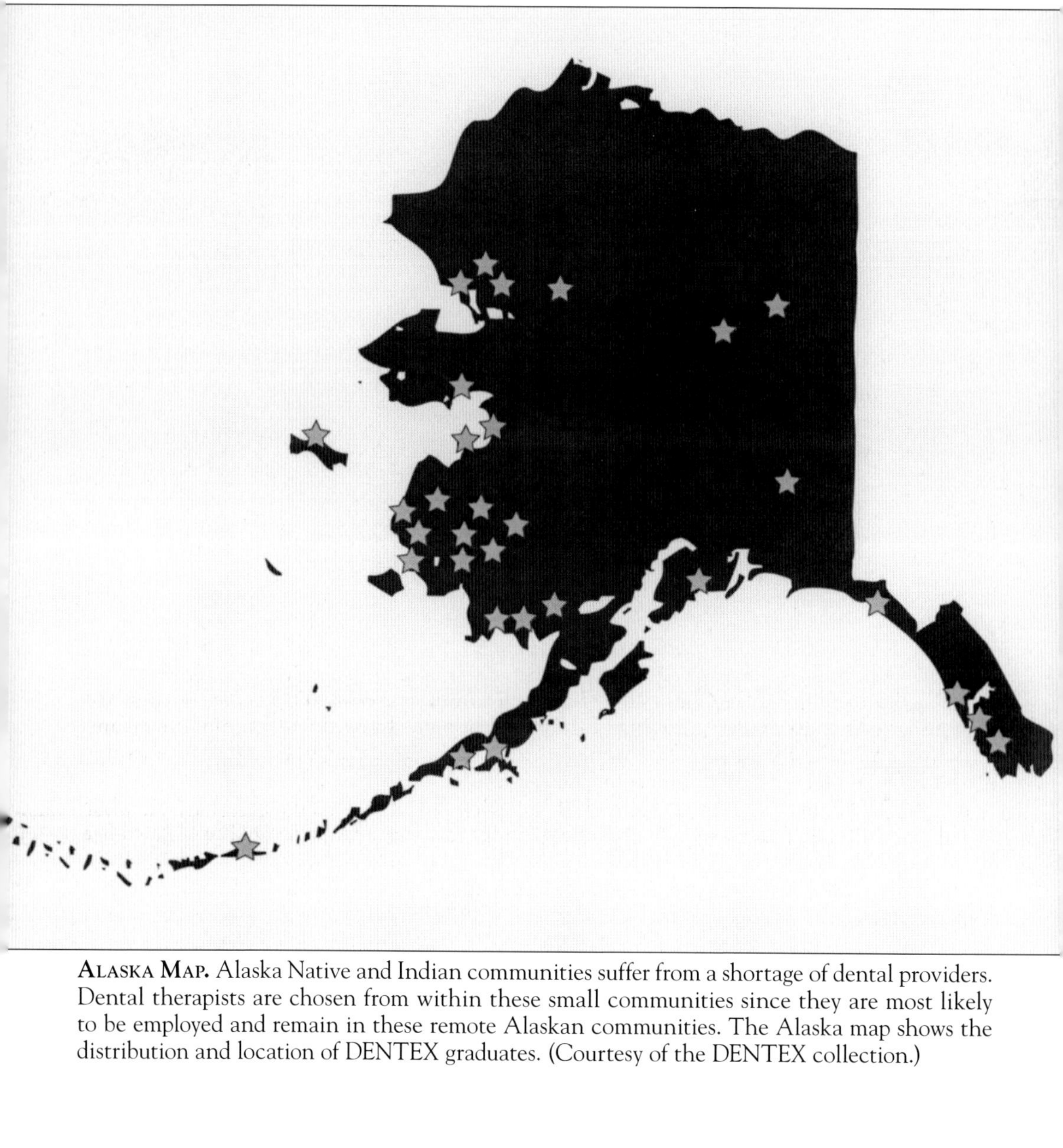

Alaska Map. Alaska Native and Indian communities suffer from a shortage of dental providers. Dental therapists are chosen from within these small communities since they are most likely to be employed and remain in these remote Alaskan communities. The Alaska map shows the distribution and location of DENTEX graduates. (Courtesy of the DENTEX collection.)

Seven

Champions, Teachers, and Leaders

From the beginning, MEDEX has had strong physician supporters and advocates, such as the program's first faculty leaders, Dr. Ray Vath and Dr. Gerald Bassett. Community physicians, including Dr. Richard Bunch in Othello and Dr. Richard Layton, then in Grandview, supported the program and served as early preceptors and advocates.

When MEDEX moved from the School of Medicine to the newly formed School of Public Health, Dean Robert Day took an active interest in the program, recruiting Dr. David Lawrence as its second director.

University of Washington Medical School faculty joined the program as adjunct faculty, and several remained throughout the years. One of these was Dr. Hugh James "Jim" Lurie, a community psychiatrist. He refined the program's behavioral medicine course by using a well-known group of Seattle actors to serve as simulated patients. Psychiatrist Dr. Nick Ward provided memorable lectures in the behavioral medicine course for many years. Pathologist Dr. Gary Goldfogel—later the medical examiner for Whatcom County—taught pathology to many classes of students. Other long-term teachers are remembered in this chapter.

Eventually, PAs themselves began to take leadership positions in the program. In 1985, Ruth Ballweg (Class 11) became program director. PA faculty and staff members, like Hahnemann graduate Henry Stoll and MEDEX administrator Jennifer Johnston, came and stayed on.

In 1994, MEDEX moved back into the School of Medicine through the leadership of Dean Philip Fialkow. Drs. John Coombs and Tom Norris helped integrate the program into the complex medical school infrastructure, which included the WWAMI regional medical program. Their strong and effective support ensured the success of MEDEX. When Dr. Paul Ramsey became dean upon the sudden death of Dr. Fialkow, he too supported MEDEX, its visibility, and its influence.

This chapter tells the story of the many MEDEX faculty and staff members who have served in MEDEX sites for more than five years. Photographs in other chapters also include current and past faculty members.

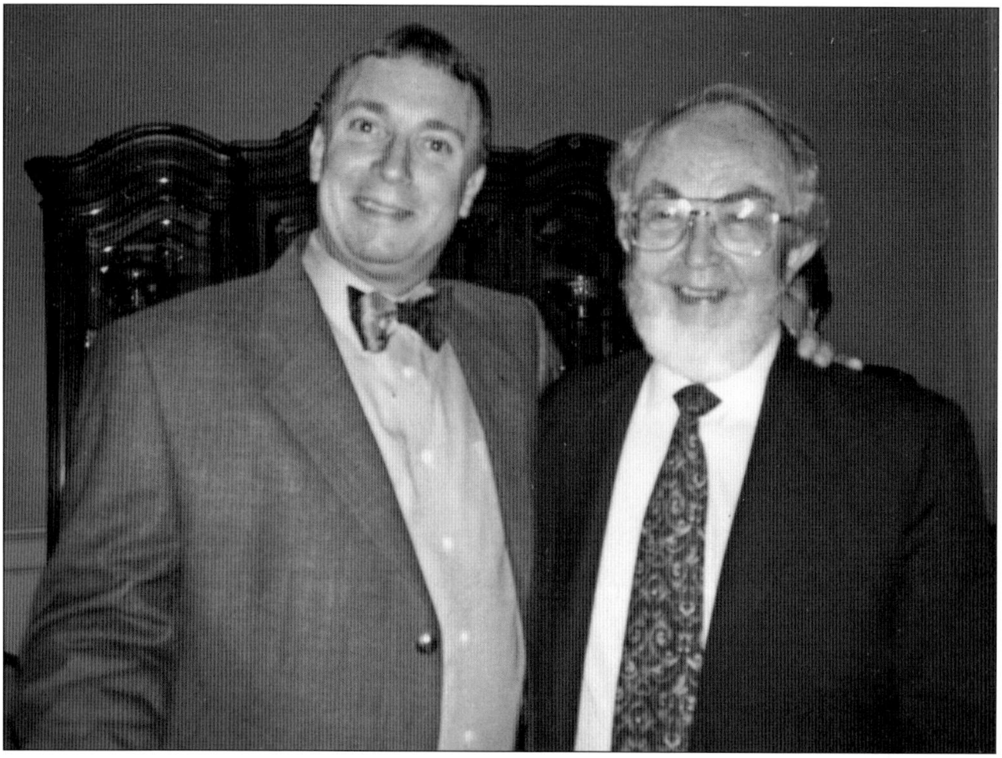

Grandview MD/PA Team. Dr. Richard Layton, right, served as preceptor for many MEDEX faculty members and for students such as Charles Hall (Class 4, left). Dr. Layton practiced for 19 years in Grandview, Washington. Later, he directed the Family Medicine Residency Program at Seattle's Providence Hospital. He served as chair of the MEDEX Physician Advisory Committee while the program was in the School of Public Health.

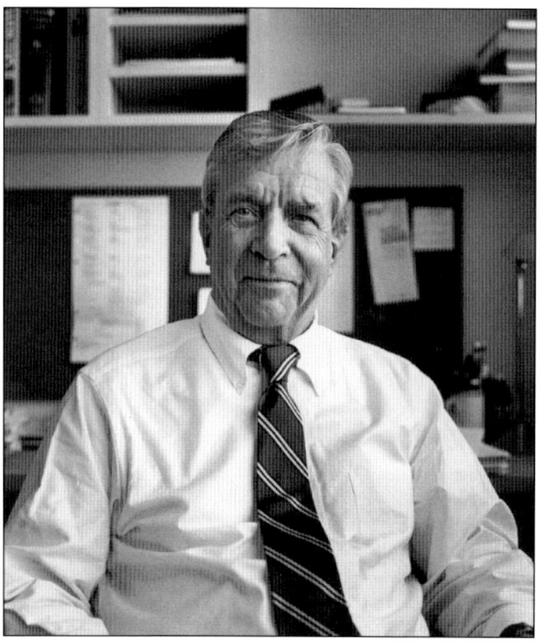

School of Public Health Dean. Dr. Robert Day, dean of the University of Washington's School of Public Health, was a strong supporter of MEDEX as it moved into the newly created school's Department of Health Services. Dr. Day recruited the second MEDEX director, Dr. David Lawrence, and also supported the creation of a self-sustaining funding category within the University of Washington, which stabilized MEDEX and saved it from closure during severe federal budget cuts in the mid-1980s.

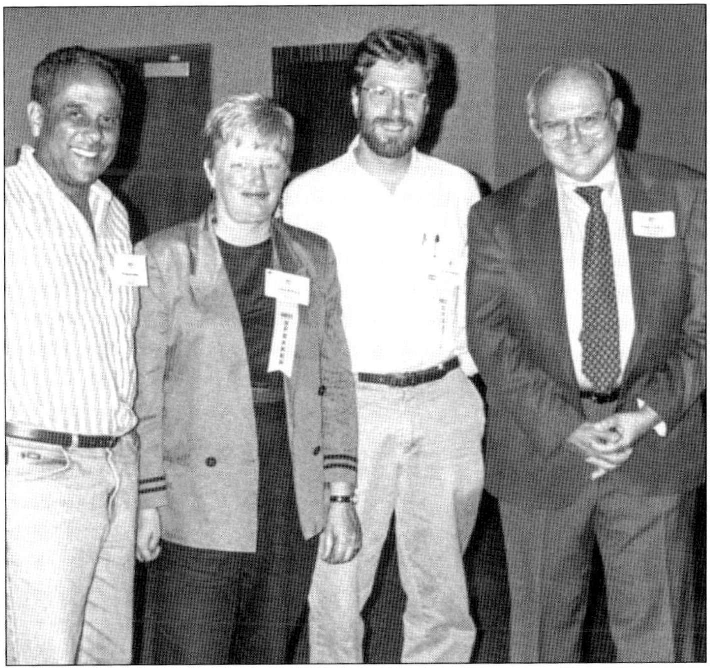

RETURN TO THE SCHOOL OF MEDICINE. In 1994, MEDEX returned to the School of Medicine through the leadership of Dean Philip Fialkow. Dr. Fialkow is shown at the far right in this photograph. Also shown are, from left to right, MEDEX founder Dr. Richard Smith; Ruth Ballweg, MEDEX program director; and Dr. Jeff Hummel, MEDEX medical director.

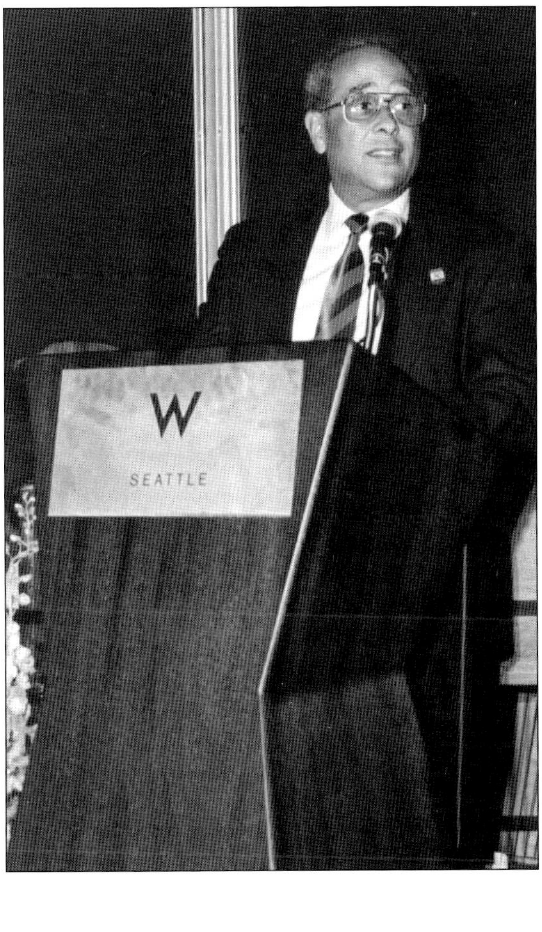

SMITH AT 30TH ANNIVERSARY. Dr. Richard Smith and his family participated in the MEDEX 30th anniversary. His presentation was inspiring and provided valuable perspective on the past and the future.

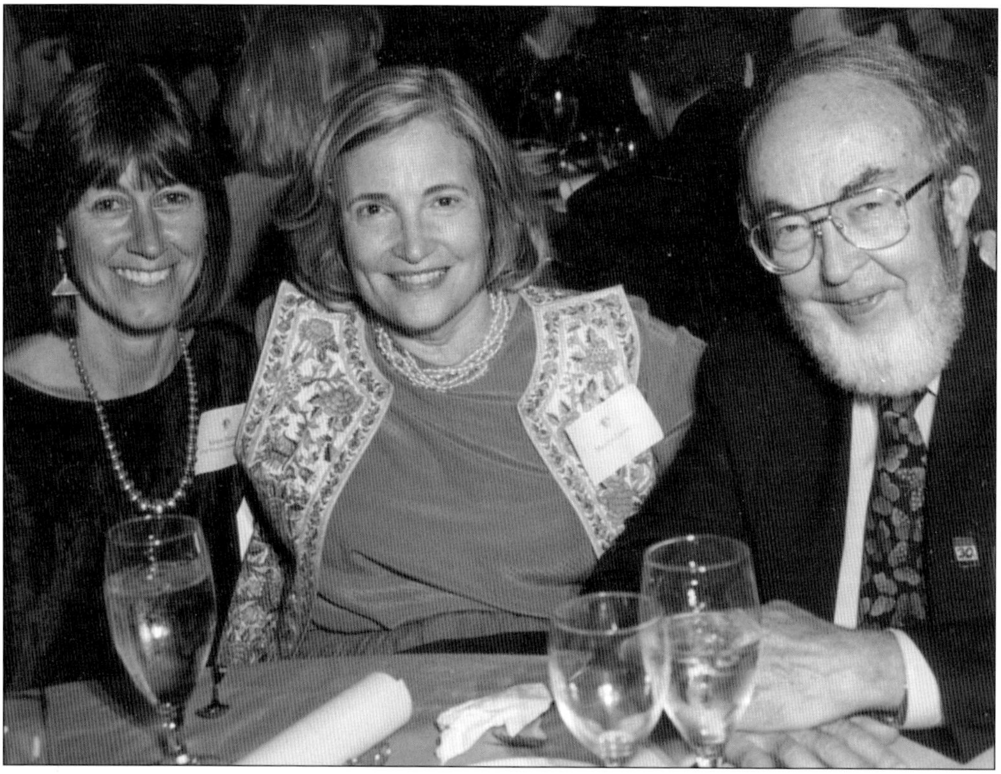

The Laytons. Dr. Richard Layton and his wife, Marilyn Layton, were honored guests at the 30th anniversary celebration and are shown here with Kirsten Thomsen, a guest from the University of New Mexico PA program. Dr. Layton is commemorated with an annual graduation award presented for "Service to Underserved Populations."

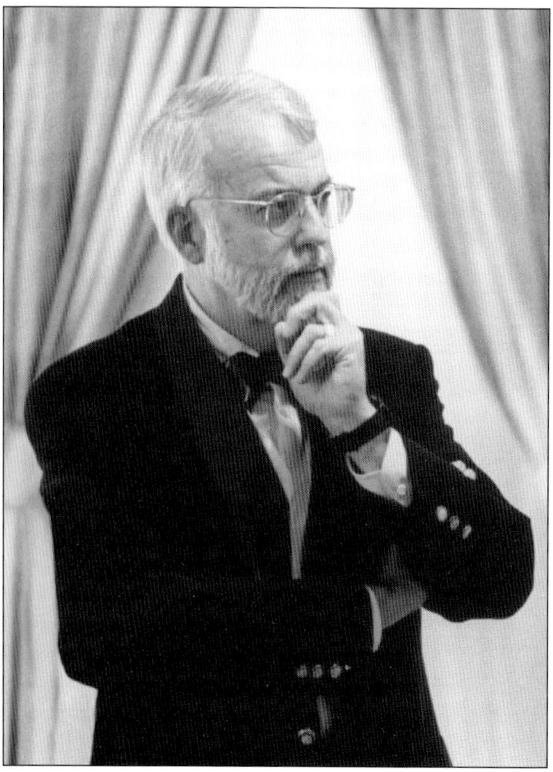

Dean of Regional Affairs. MEDEX was initially assigned to the Department of Medical Education as its academic home. However, the program's main reporting function was to Dr. John Coombs, then the dean of regional affairs. Dr. Coombs facilitated the integration of MEDEX into the School of Medicine infrastructure, including introduction to leaders and clinical department chairs and direct representation on major School of Medicine committees. (Courtesy of the University of Washington, Office of Graduate Medical Education, Dean of Medicine.)

Founding Site Director. Barbara Gunter-Flynn (Class 12) was the founding site director for both the Yakima and Spokane sites. Barbara's background included service as a Coast Guard corpswoman and later in leadership roles at the Department of Corrections and at Group Health. Here, she is shown with John Yerxa (Class 18).

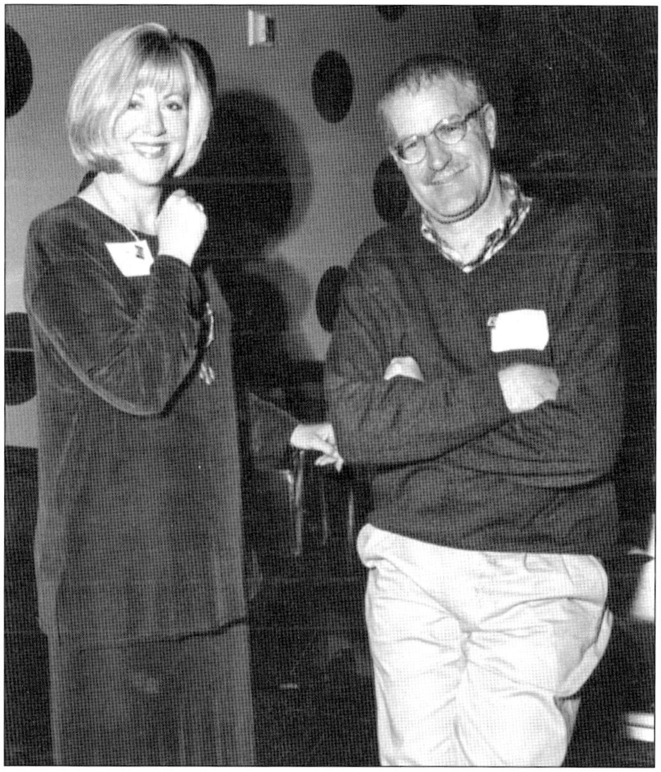

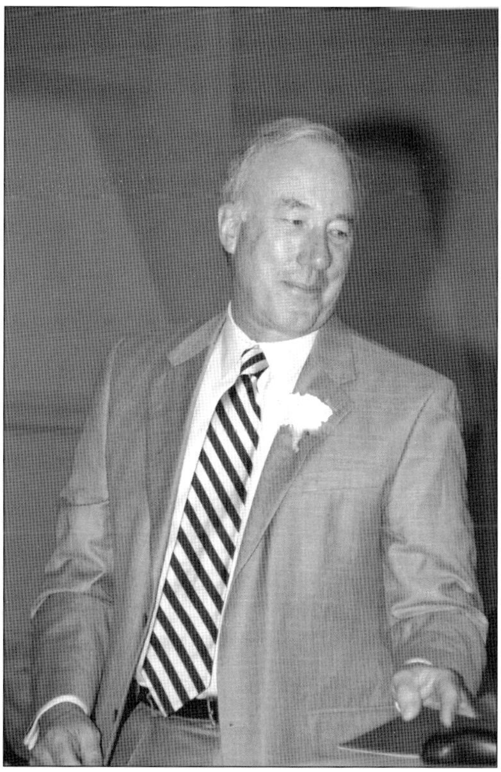

Family Medicine Leader. The School of Medicine leader, Dr. Tom Norris, was also assigned to work with MEDEX on transition issues. He provided valuable advice on implementation and business considerations. Later chair of the Department of Family Medicine, Dr. Norris provided the leadership for MEDEX to be transferred into family medicine.

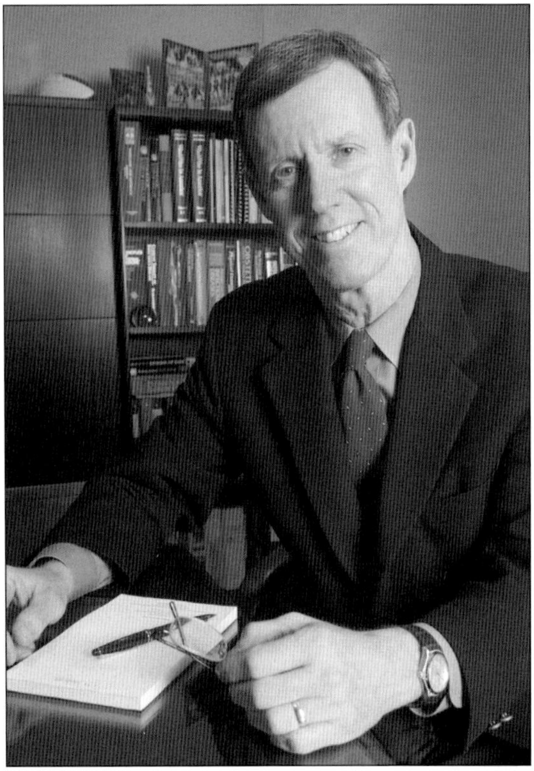

Dean Ramsey. Dr. Paul Ramsey succeeded Dr. Fialkow as dean of the School of Medicine. Dr. Ramsey has provided strong, enthusiastic support for the MEDEX program and for expanded utilization of physician assistants within the School of Medicine clinic systems. As a personal touch, Dr. Ramsey visits Seattle classes on the first day of lectures; his welcome speech has become a popular tradition. (Courtesy of Clare McLean, University of Washington School of Medicine.)

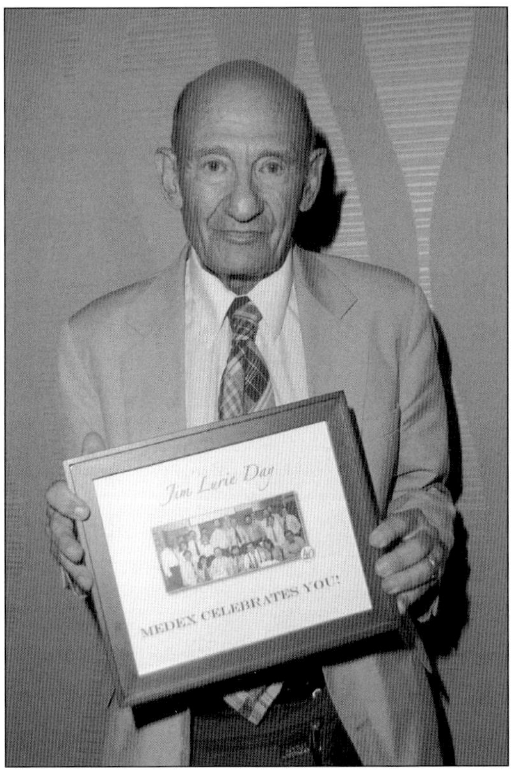

Psychiatrist Lurie. Community Psychiatrist Dr. Jim Lurie is one of the physicians who had the greatest impact on MEDEX—and MEDEX students—over time. Dr. Lurie joined MEDEX in 1974 and retired in 2009 after teaching students at all MEDEX sites.

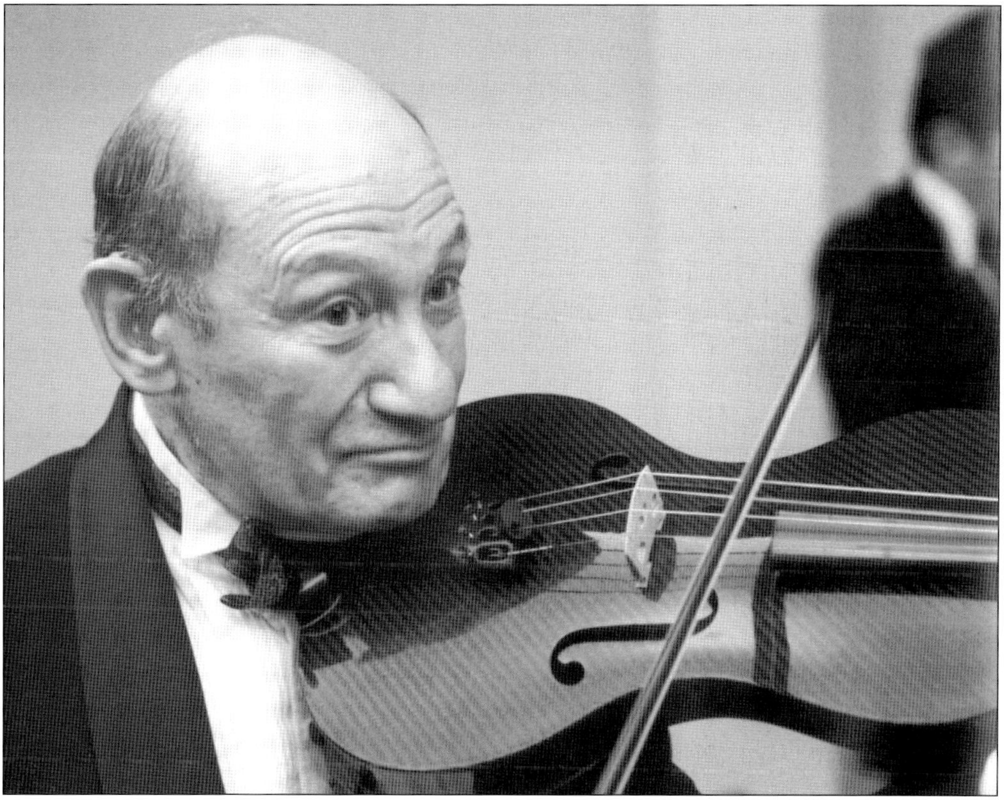

Lurie the Artist. Music and art were some of Dr. Lurie's greatest pleasures. He loved chamber music and played with many informal groups of music lovers throughout his life. He also personally hosted many musical rehearsals and events for his friends. (Courtesy of the Lurie Family.)

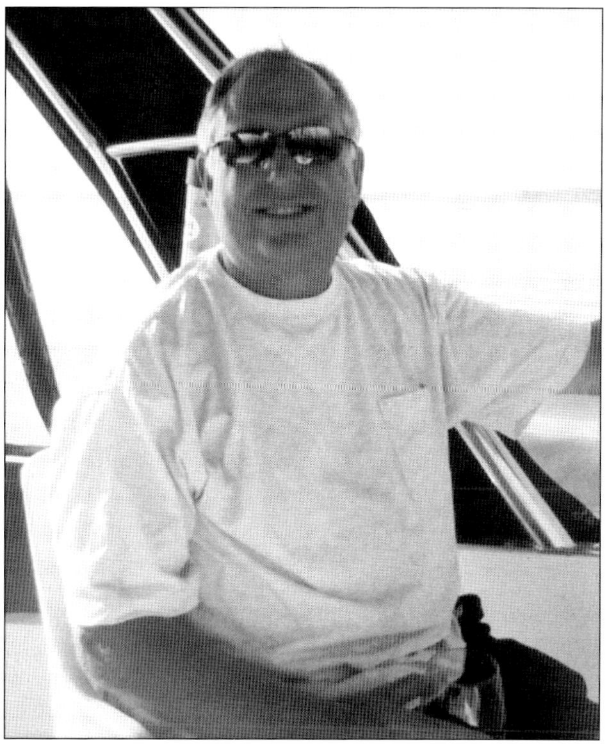

Pathologist Goldfogel. Dr. Gary Goldfogel made the difficult concepts of pathology and pathophysiology come alive in the MEDEX pathology course. Since moving away from Seattle, Dr. Goldfogel is the medical examiner in Whatcom County and has served in major leadership positions in the Washington State Medical Association. (Courtesy of Gary Goldfogel.)

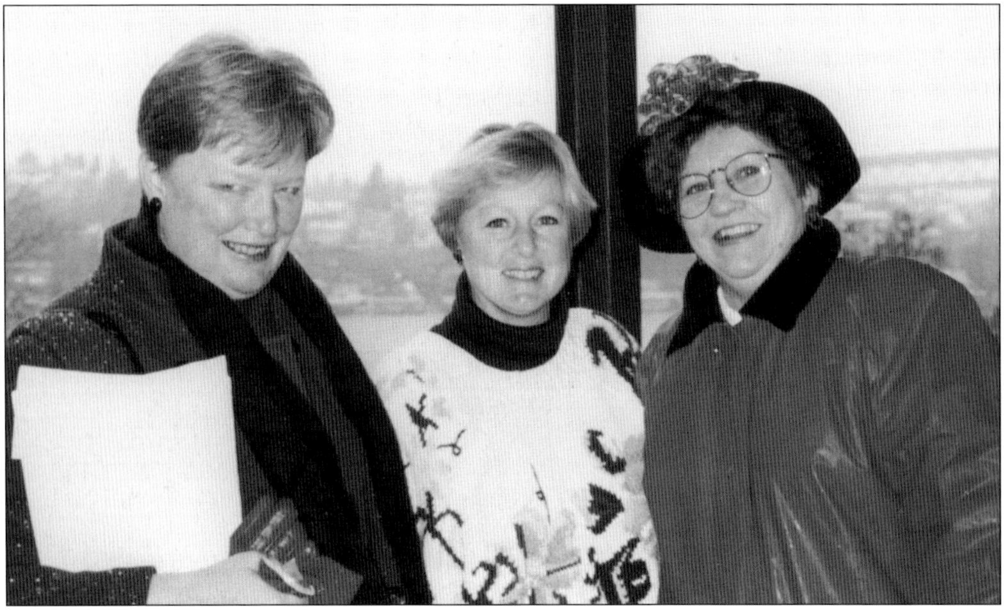

MEDEX Women Leaders. Strong women leaders have been important for the MEDEX program. Program administrator Jennifer Johnston (center) and program director Ruth Ballweg (left) partnered with each other for years to develop and expand the MEDEX program. Pictured with them is Jo Asplin (right), a graduate of the child health associate program and course director of the maternal child health course.

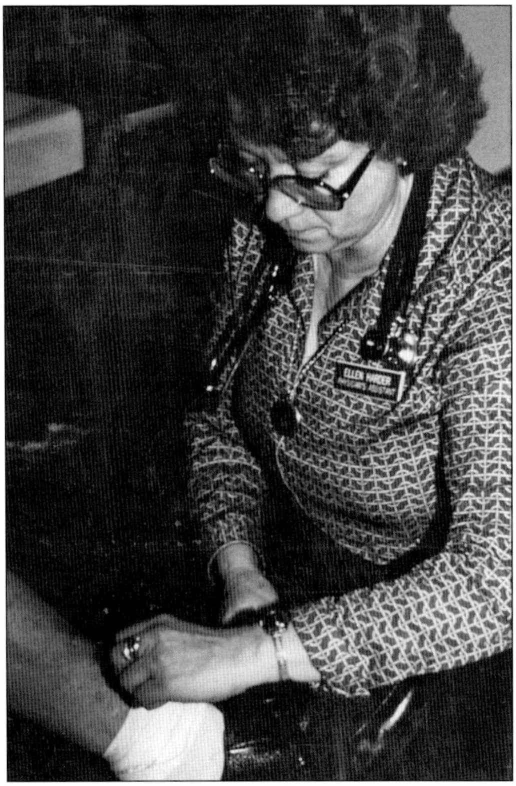

MEDEX Clinical Coordinator. Ellen Harder (Class 12) served as MEDEX clinical coordinator until her retirement. A member of MEDEX Class 12, Harder practiced primary care in a community health center in Yakima, at the Pike Market Clinic, and in Group Health before joining MEDEX. As clinical coordinator, she developed new clinical sites throughout the WWAMI region. A strong advocate for students from nontraditional backgrounds, Harder was beloved by many. She later served on the Medical Quality Assurance Commission, the National Commission on Certification of Physician Assistants, and was the PA representative to the Federation of State Medical Boards.

Faculty Member Terry Scott. Terry Scott (Class 25) has served in both the didactic and clinical phases of the MEDEX curriculum and practiced in the family medicine residency. Scott became program director in 2014 and overall leader of the MEDEX program on July 1, 2015.

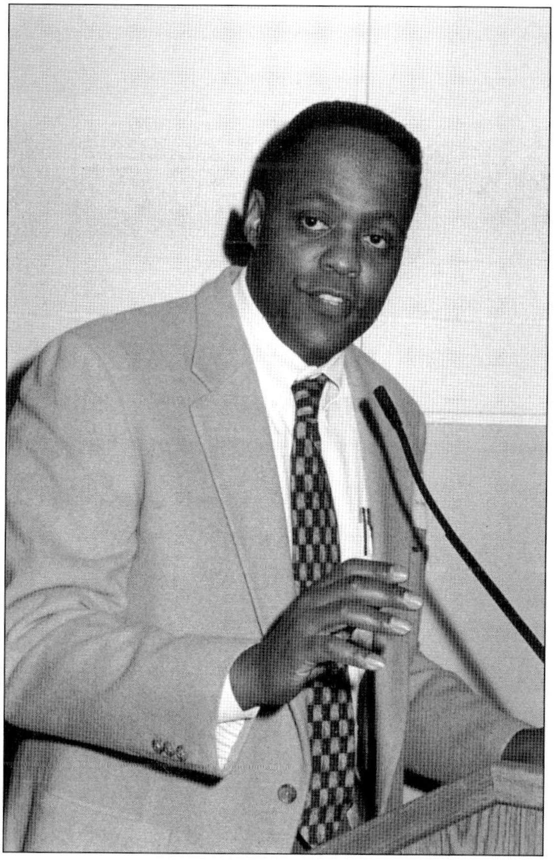

Service and Joy. Doreen Blomstrand (Class 17) stands on Ellen Harder's right, at Harder's retirement party. Blomstrand worked as an EMT and medical assistant in Alaska, Micronesia, and in Cambodian refugee camps. Faced with the sudden loss of her husband, she applied to MEDEX and later joined the faculty. In her MEDEX application, she summarized her career in a simple but profound statement: "Working with people in service is my joy."

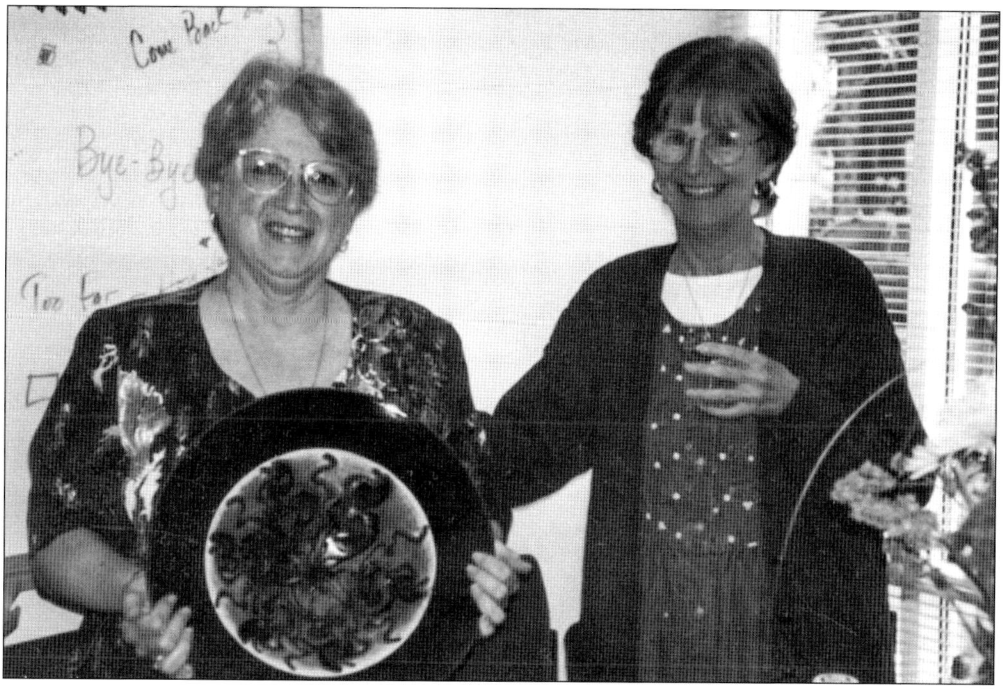

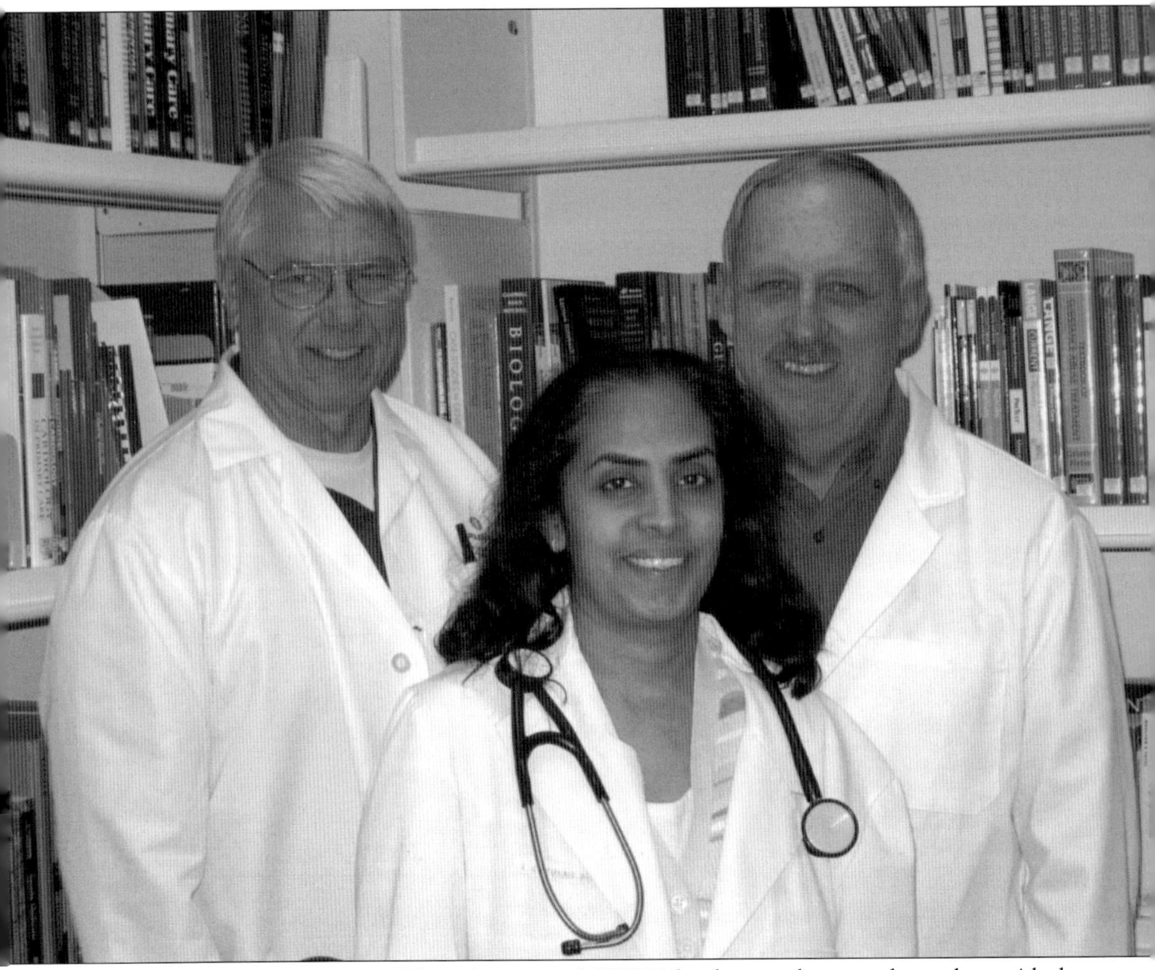

Seattle Faculty Members. Three long-term MEDEX faculty members are shown here. Alaskan Bill Plummer (left) trained and worked as a PA in the military. Plummer served as the MEDEX rural clinic coordinator. Amee Naidu (center) specialized in internal medicine and geriatrics before joining MEDEX on the didactic faculty. Henry Stoll (right) graduated from the Hahnemann (now Drexel) PA program and has held many didactic teaching roles at MEDEX. He served as the first site coordinator for the Tacoma MEDEX site.

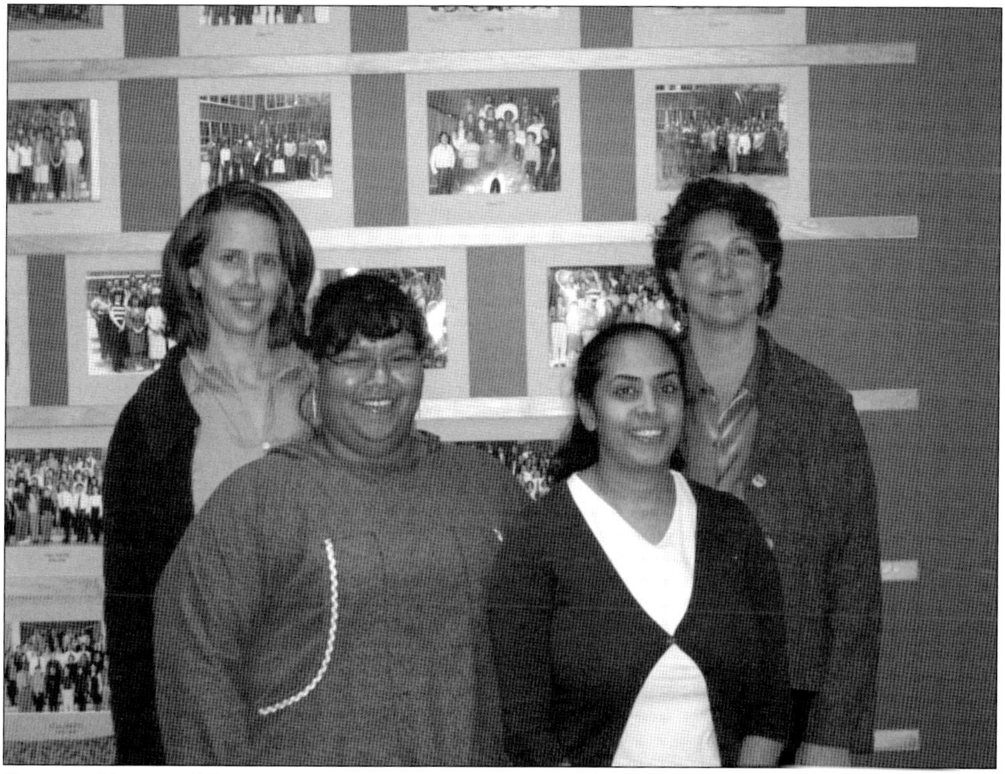

Seattle Faculty Members. MEDEX didactic faculty members have included (from left to right) Alexa Gregory Martin, Teresa Flores, Amee Naidu, and Dianna Wachtel.

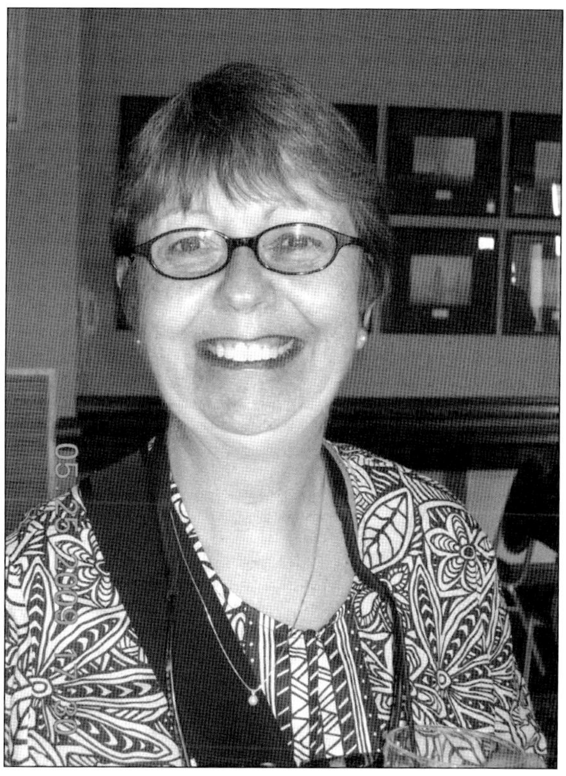

ER Faculty Member. A Stanford PA graduate, Kaye Kvam served as the codirector of the emergency medicine residency at LA County Hospital before moving to the Pacific Northwest. Kvam is regarded as an amazing classroom teacher who regularly uses pranks, costumes, and silly situations to make her point in a wide range of lectures.

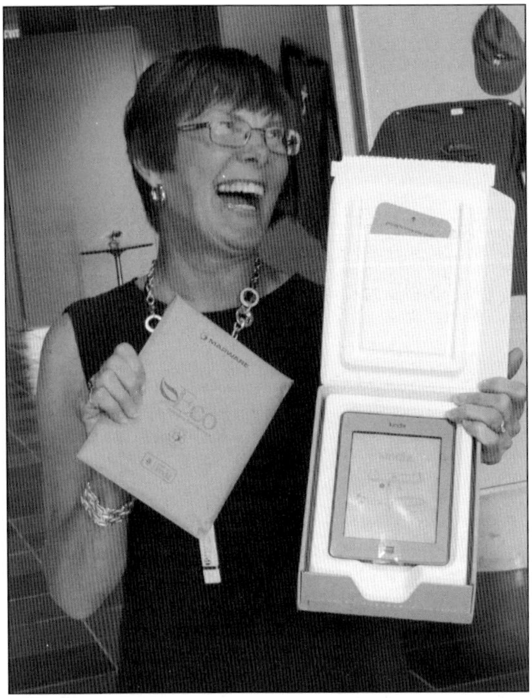

Spokane Faculty Member. NP Sharon Moses served in the Air Force for many years, then joined the first MEDEX faculty in Spokane. She was a clinical coordinator, as well as a popular didactic lecturer. After this party honoring her so-called retirement, Moses tackled projects in clinical and didactic support for MEDEX Anchorage.

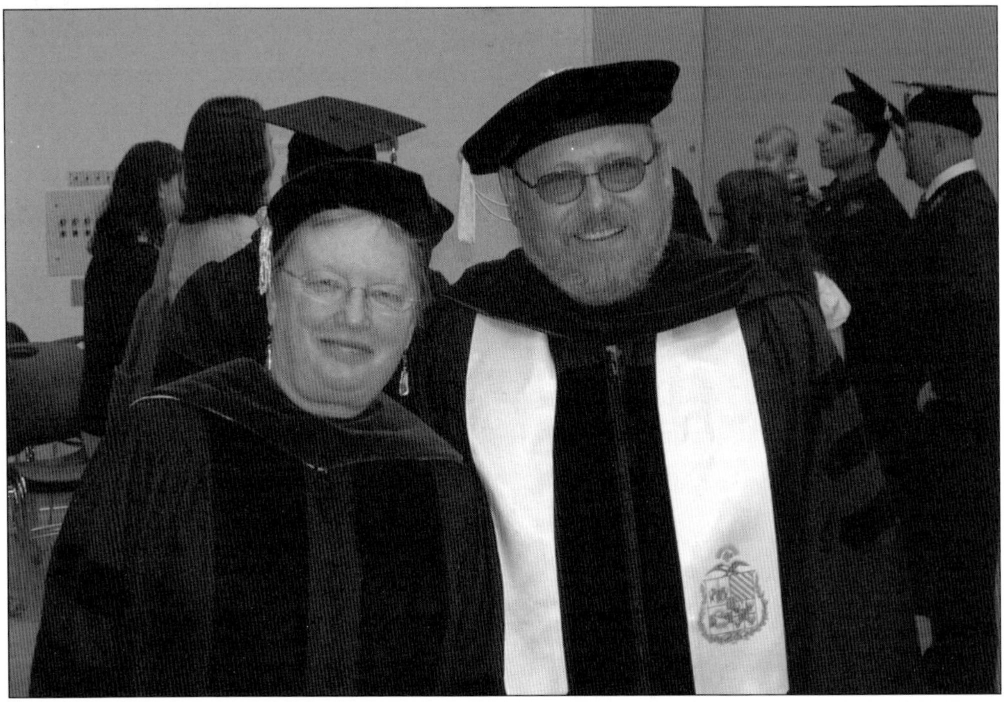

Spokane Faculty Member. Former Air Force PA Don Coerver is shown here with Ruth Ballweg at the first master's degree graduation in Spokane. Coerver was a founding faculty member for the Spokane site and has received many teaching accolades throughout his career. His background includes special training and extensive practice in the specialty of orthopedics. While at MEDEX, he completed his doctorate at Gonzaga University.

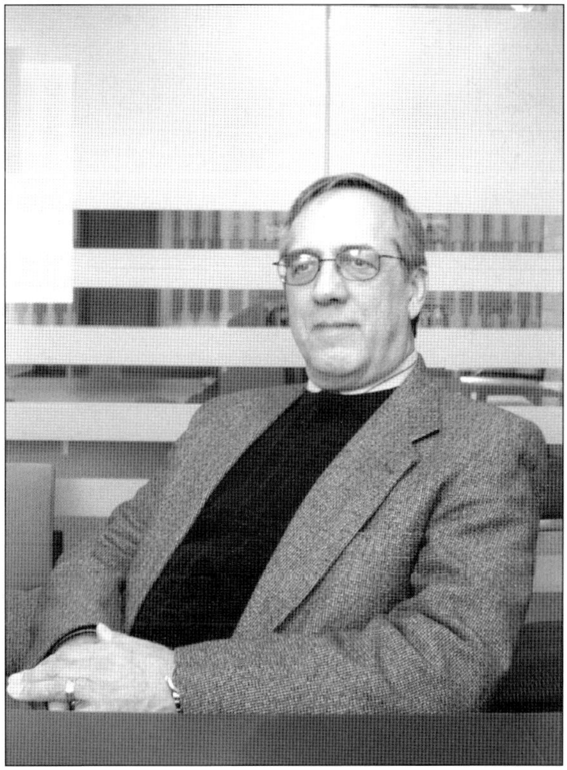

Spokane PA Leader. Steve Meltzer, a graduate of the Duke PA program, led the Spokane site from 2004 until his retirement in 2013. After practicing primary care in rural Eastern Washington, Meltzer became the director of the Eastern Washington Area Health Education Center, where he led rural health advocacy and policy activities. He also served as president of the Washington Academy of Physician Assistants.

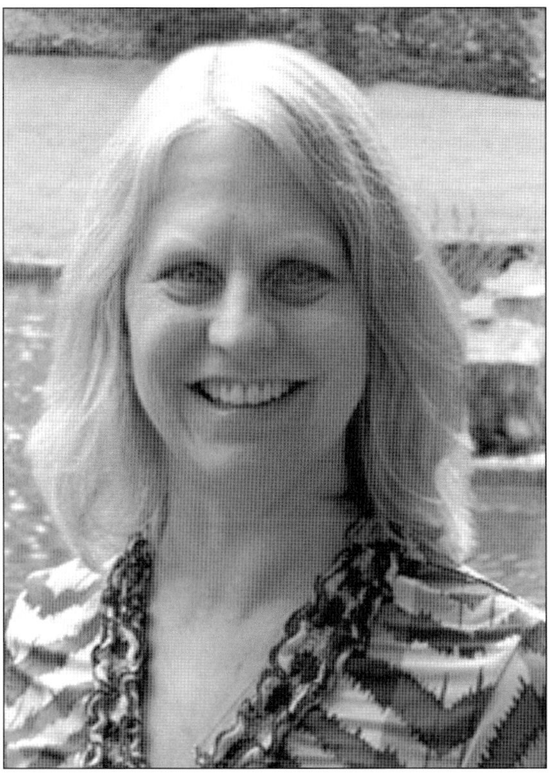

Medical Director. Medical director Dr. Linda Vorvick is a family physician who worked in the Providence Medical System prior to joining MEDEX. From May 1, 2014, through June 2015, Dr. Vorvick served as interim section chief for MEDEX.

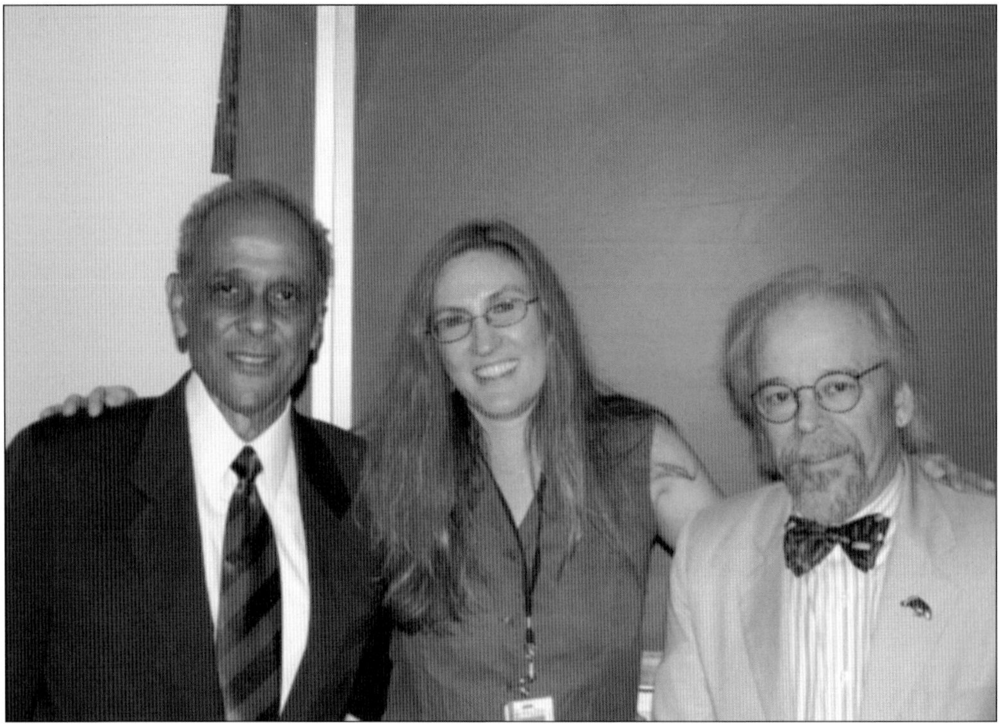

Smith and Faculty Members. Dr. Richard Smith is pictured with Keren Wick and Gino Gianola at a MEDEX celebration. As the MEDEX director of graduate education and research, Wick played a major role in the development and implementation of the MEDEX master's degree curriculum.

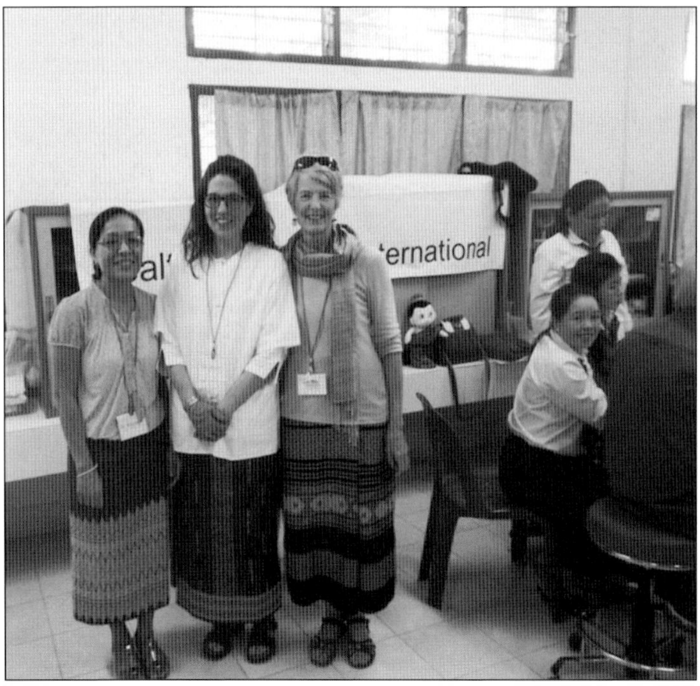

Health Leadership International. From left to right are Khampho Ohno (Class 43); Alicia Quella, MEDEX Spokane coordinator; and Susan "Reba" McIntyre. McIntyre heads the MEDEX master's in global health course. They are pictured in Luan Prabang, Laos, as representatives of Health Leadership International. Khampho is leading the development of a Lao PA program. (Courtesy Susan McIntyre.)

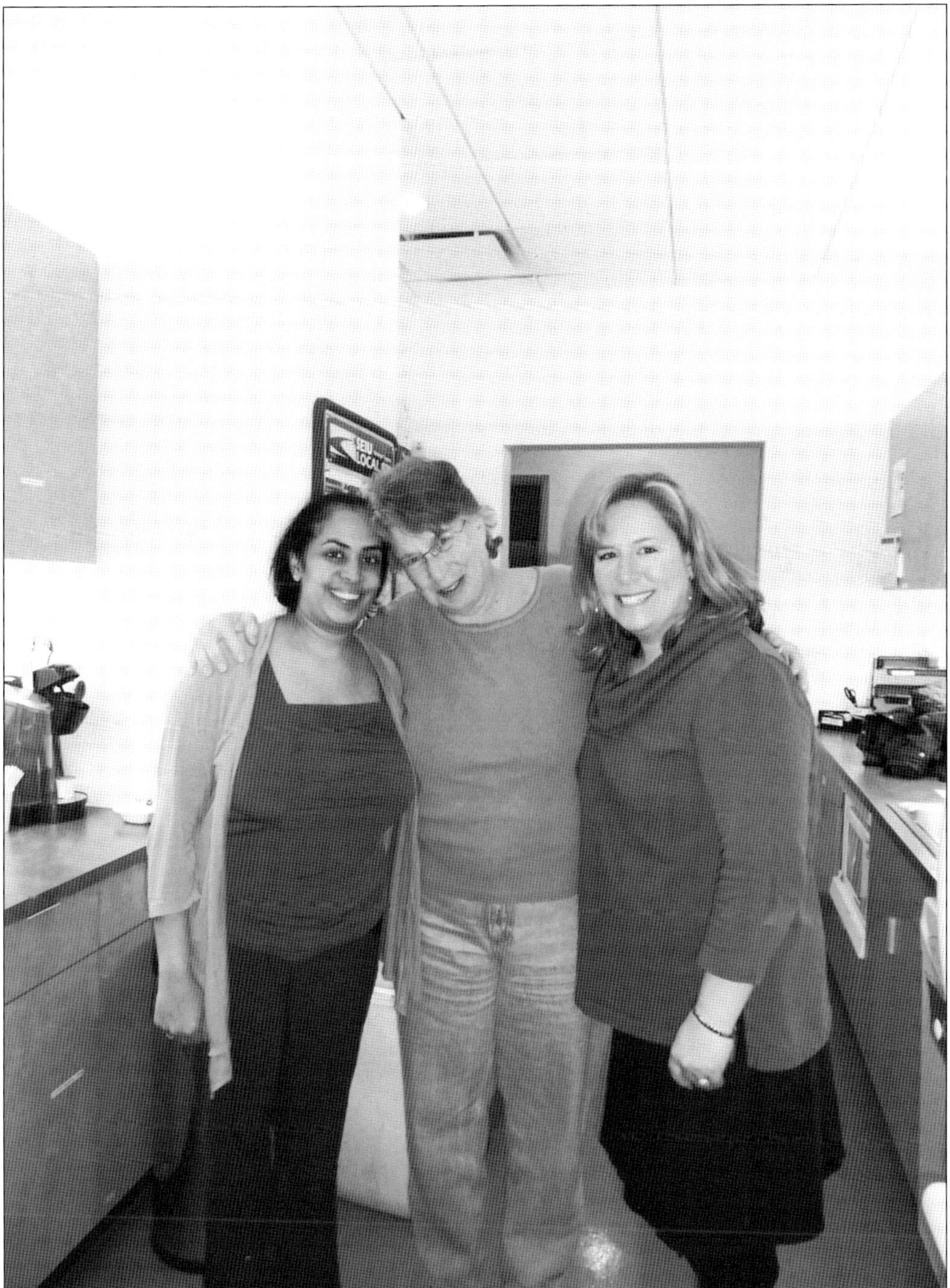

Didactic Faculty Members. From left to right, three didactic faculty members, Amee Naidu, Lois Thetford, and Kira Vader, are shown in the MEDEX kitchen. Naidu is specifically known and appreciated for her special support of students preparing for the certification exam. Thetford (Class 14), a recipient of a Jefferson Award for her community service, is seen as a strong voice for social justice and advocacy. Vader (Class 27) has first contact with entering students through the online Anatomy and Physiology course.

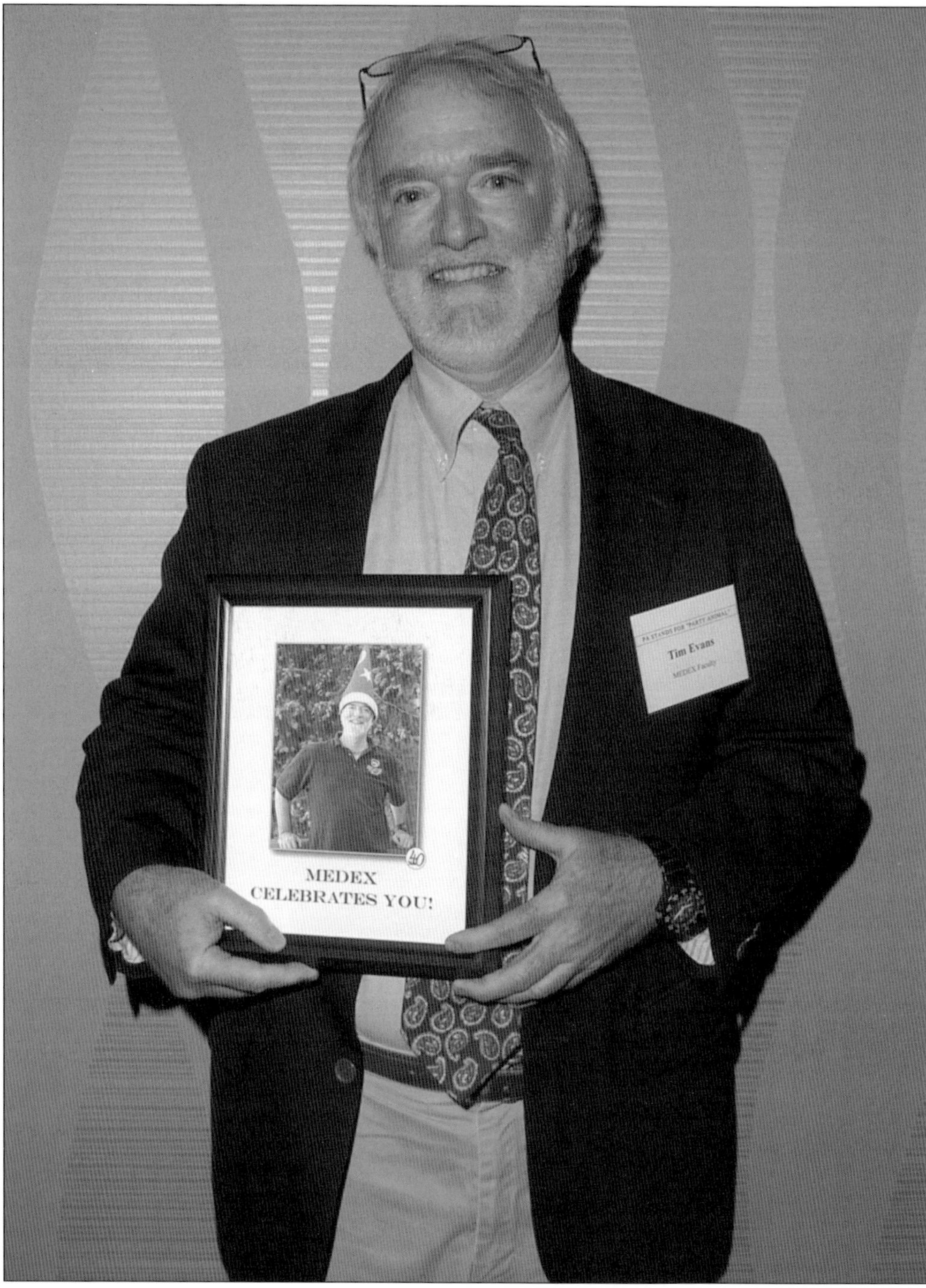

Dr. Evans. Senior medical director Dr. Tim Evans teaches medicine topics across all four MEDEX sites. MEDEX graduates also benefit from his outstanding lectures at Continuing Medical Education conferences throughout the region. Dr. Evans has served as the American College of Physicians' representative to the Accreditation Review Commission on Education for the Physician Assistant (ARC-PA) and to the National Commission on Certification of Physician Assistants. (NCCPA)

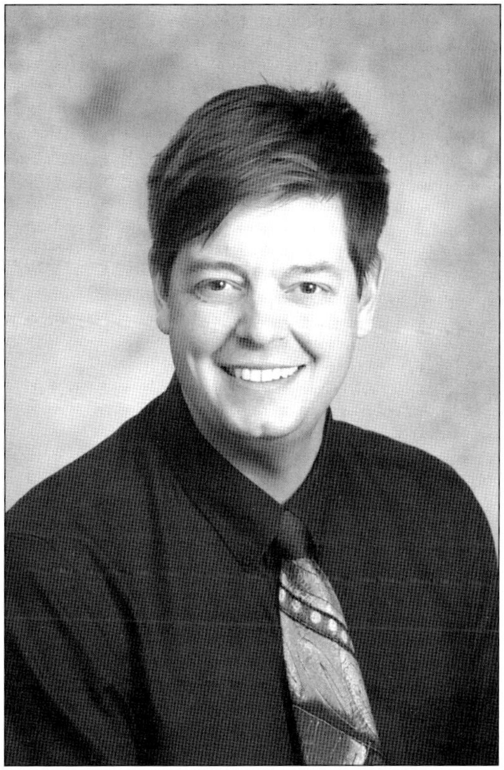

University of Washington Internal Medicine Teacher. Dr. Chris Knight, a University of Washington internist, began his involvement with MEDEX early in his faculty career. Teaching the most difficult and complex cardiology content, Dr. Knight engages the students in active and participatory learning. Dr. Knight is coleader of the academic medicine/specialty practice pathway in the master's degree curriculum.

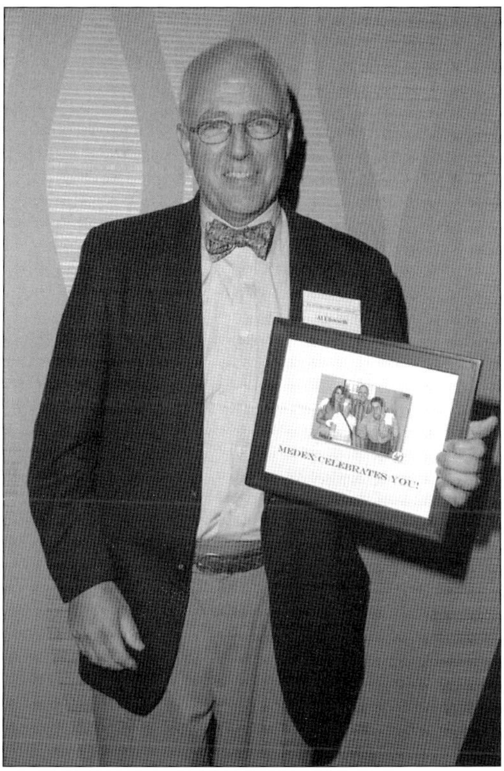

Pharmacology PA. Allan Ellsworth (Class 34), PharmD, began teaching in the MEDEX Pharmacology Course in 1982 as a faculty member in the Department of Family Medicine. He later enrolled in MEDEX and became a PA himself. Ellsworth practices as a PA in the rural community of Sultan, Washington, and continues to teach at MEDEX.

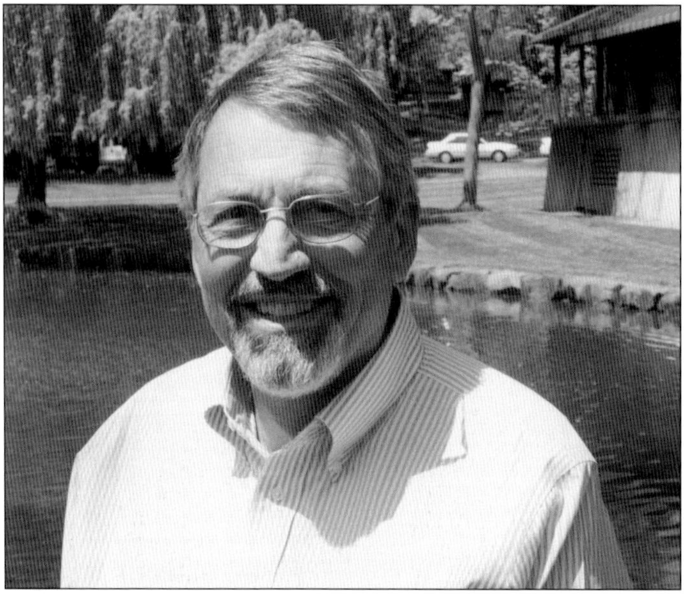

Master's Program Faculty Member. Bill Tozier, PhD, PA-C, joined the MEDEX faculty after serving in senior leadership in the US Army. A graduate of the Duke University PA program, Tozier is the recipient of the AAPA Veteran's Caucus Military PA of the Year Award. Tozier served as the program director for the Interservice PA program. He is the leader of the public health/ prevention pathway in the master's degree curriculum and serves as an advisor for student research.

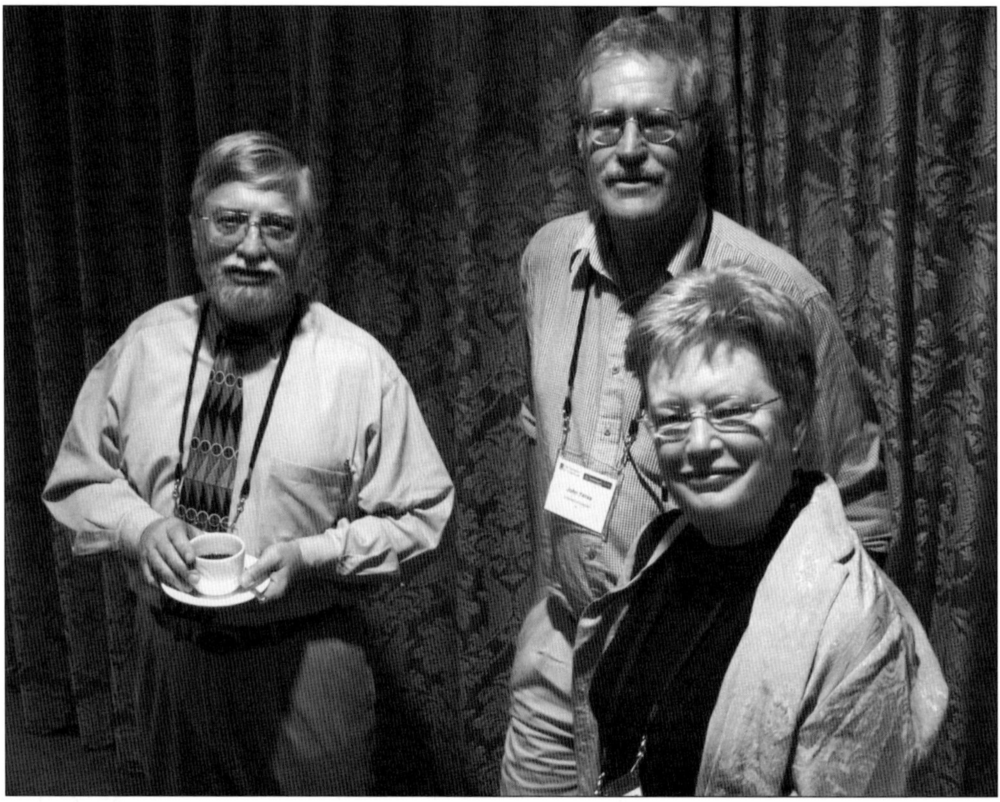

National PA Researcher. A highly recognized researcher and clinician, Dr. Roderick Hooker is shown in 2005 with John Yerxa (Class 18) and Ruth Ballweg at the first Australian health workforce conference to consider the introduction of PAs. At MEDEX, Dr. Hooker taught research methodology and served as a master's capstone advisor. A graduate of the St. Louis University PA program, he practiced in the Kaiser Permanente system as a veterans administrator.

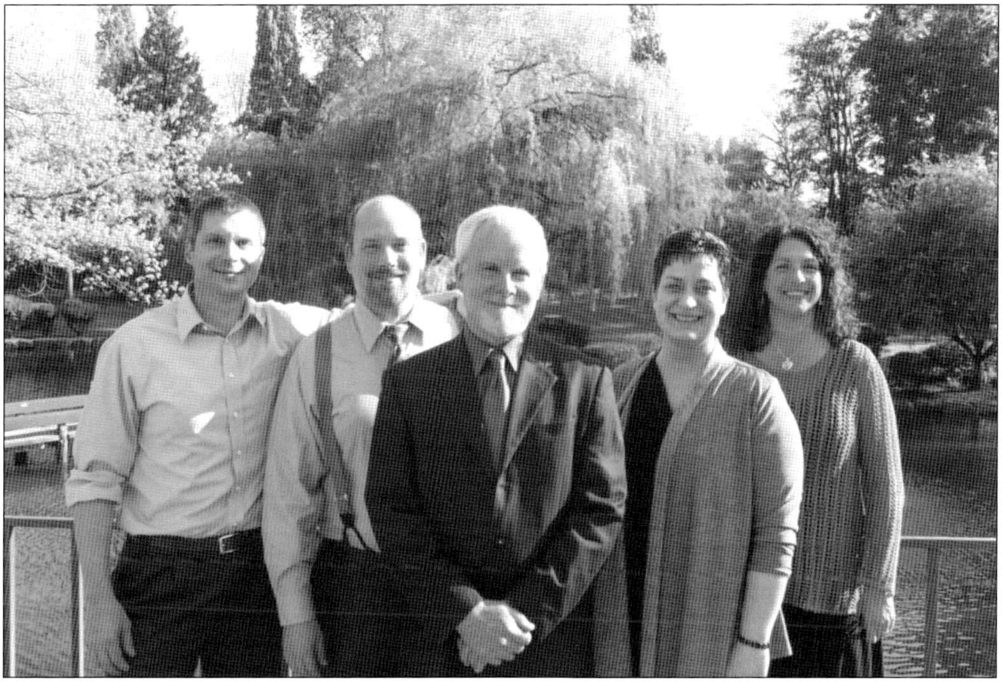

Admissions. The MEDEX admissions team works together to actively recruit and select a diverse student body composed of individuals with significant health-care experience. Shown here in 2011 are, from left to right, Ky Haverkamp, Tony Skaggs, Tim Quigley, Mariah Kindle, and Dianna Wachtel.

Alaska Faculty and Staff. The Anchorage MEDEX site was opened to its first students in 2009. Anchorage faculty included Denise Coslett, Pat Hensch, Ashley Marquardt, John Riley, Carol Chambers, and Rick Fradl. Other photographs of Alaska faculty members appear in Chapter 9.

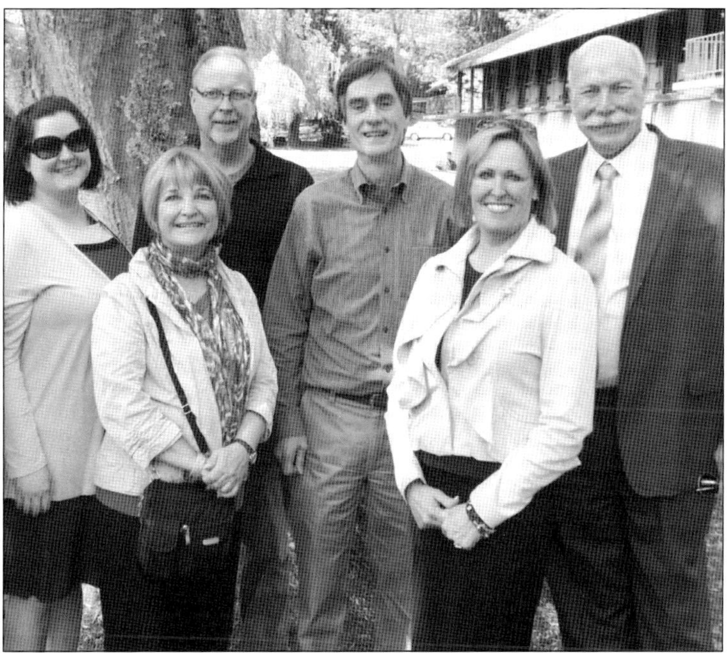

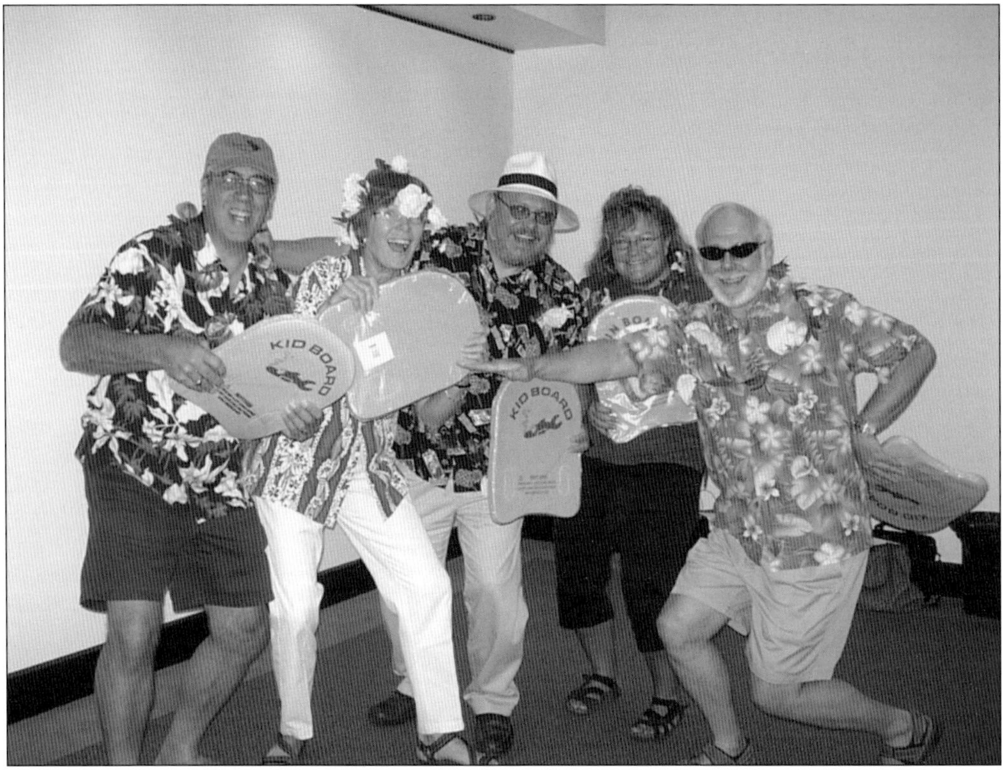

SPOKANE FACULTY. Demonstrating that "PA stands for Party Animal," the Spokane faculty is shown demonstrating their best beach clothing and surfing moves.

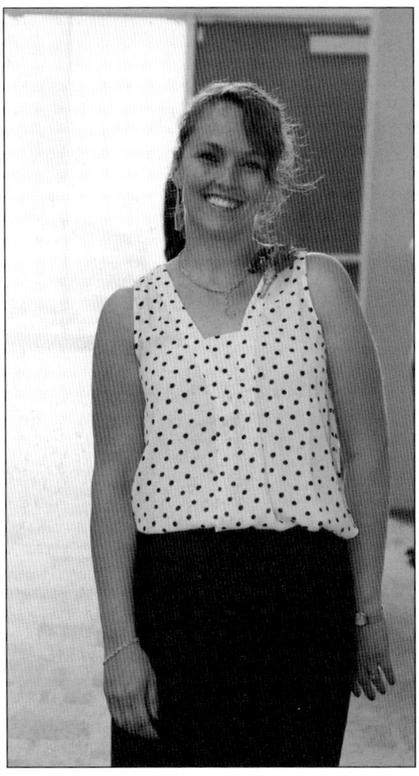

TACOMA LEADERSHIP. Vanessa Bester, PA-C, MPAS, graduated from the University of Florida program. Bester's experience includes HIV primary care through the National Health Service Corps and cardiology with the US Army in Germany. In Tacoma, she works with medical programs at Madigan Army Medical Center. She became the Tacoma site director in July 2015.

Eight

DECENTRALIZED TRAINING

From the beginning, MEDEX saw itself as a regional rather than as a state-specific program. Originally housed in the University of Washington's School of Medicine, MEDEX was one of several federally funded health workforce innovations during Lyndon Johnson's "Great Society" and was designed to increase health-care access in the Pacific Northwest. Simultaneously, family medicine and nurse practitioner programs were created at the University of Washington. At one point, consideration was given to create a new School of Primary Care to include family physicians, nurse practitioners, and MEDEX. Most notably, the WAMI medical education region was created to enable the University of Washington School of Medicine to serve as the medical school for the states of Washington, Alaska, Montana, and Idaho. Later, when Wyoming joined the group, the acronym became WWAMI. As a regional medical program, WWAMI created opportunities for each state to purchase slots in the University of Washington School of Medicine with a curriculum designed to return new doctors to their home states. In addition to educating medical students, WWAMI has served as the foundation for a number of regional medical-related programs including a family medicine residency network, a regional medical referral system, and continuing medical education.

Although MEDEX has never received WWAMI funding, it has been closely tied with WWAMI programs and initiatives. Before there was a rapid expansion of PA programs in the 1990s, MEDEX served as the only program for the WWAMI states plus Oregon and Hawaii. In 1993, MEDEX began its own decentralized process by establishing classroom sites first in Sitka, Alaska, and then in Yakima (1993) and Spokane, Washington (1997); Anchorage, Alaska (2008); and finally Tacoma, Washington (2013). In Sitka, MEDEX first developed its decentralized model as a strategy to keep rural students closer to their home communities. The Sitka and Yakima sites eventually closed as MEDEX developed more efficient and formal sites by partnering with other academic settings.

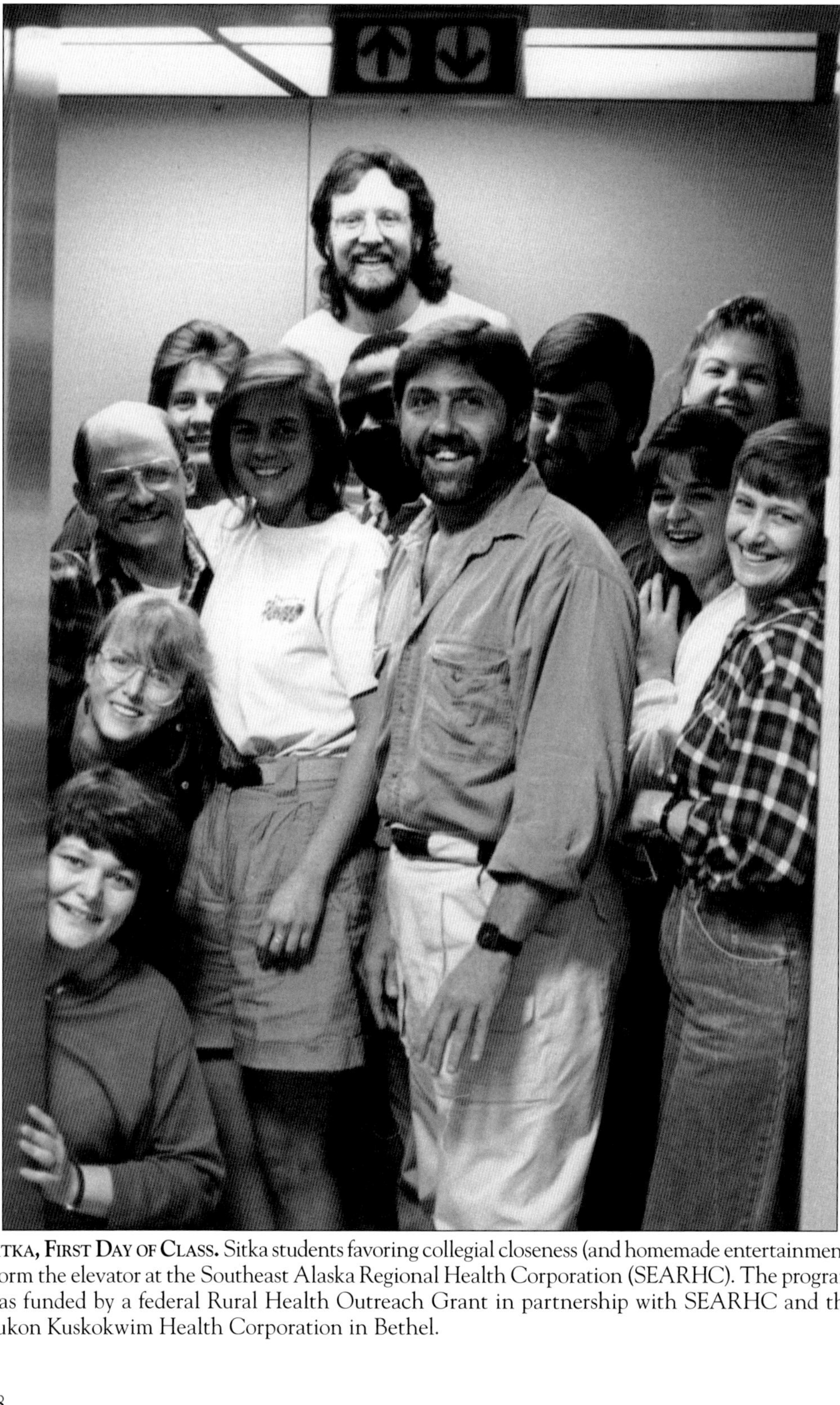

Sitka, First Day of Class. Sitka students favoring collegial closeness (and homemade entertainment) storm the elevator at the Southeast Alaska Regional Health Corporation (SEARHC). The program was funded by a federal Rural Health Outreach Grant in partnership with SEARHC and the Yukon Kuskokwim Health Corporation in Bethel.

Sitka on the Air. Howard Straker, MPH, PA-C, taught as lecturer and advisor for the MEDEX Sitka satellite in 1993–1994, with some air time at this Sitka radio station. A Yale program graduate, he worked at the Harlem PA program before joining Sitka. He later completed his master's in public health at the University of North Carolina. He is now assistant professor and director of community medicine at the George Washington University PA program.

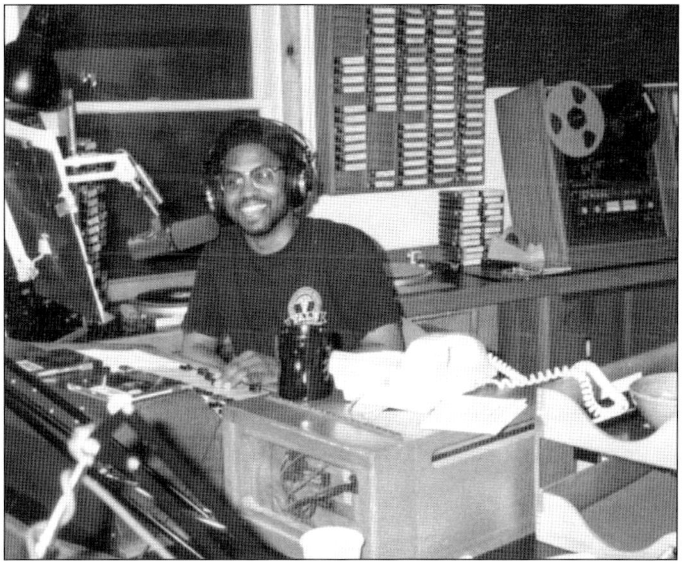

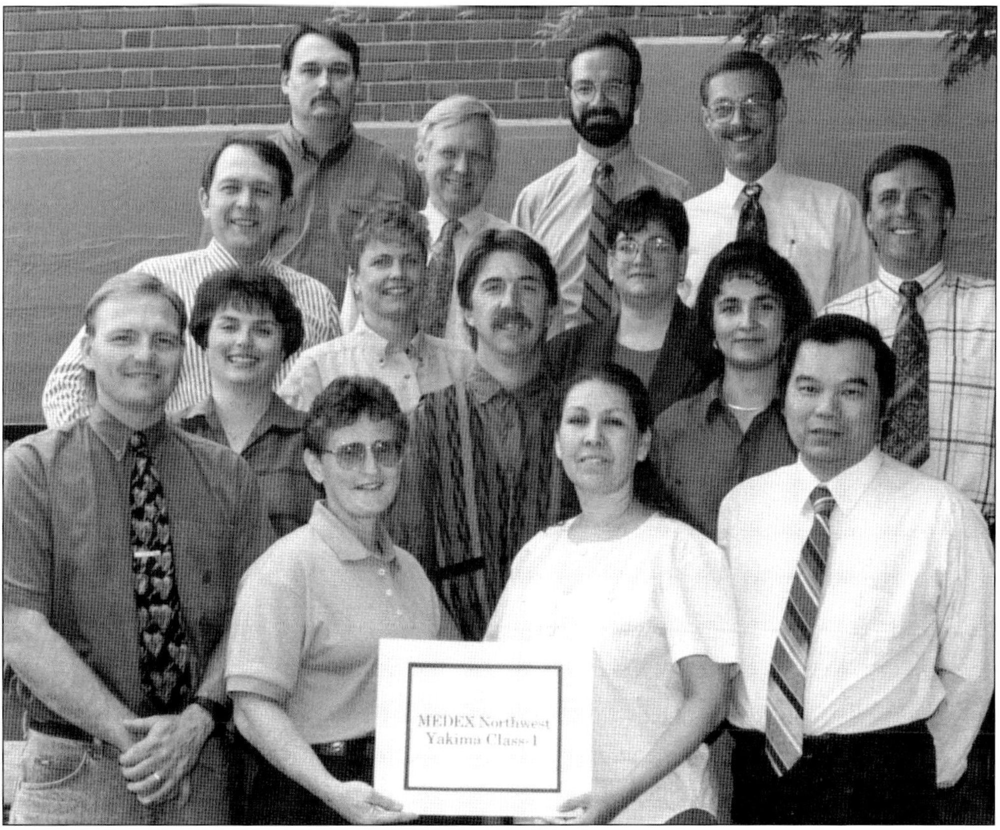

First Yakima Class. MEDEX was quickly able to apply what it learned about decentralized training in Sitka to a new site in Yakima in 1996. With strong support from a community advisory board, the initial class was composed almost entirely of students from Central and Eastern Washington. Led by Barbara Gunter-Flynn, the Yakima program initially used classrooms in both Yakima hospitals as a strategy to promote the new program.

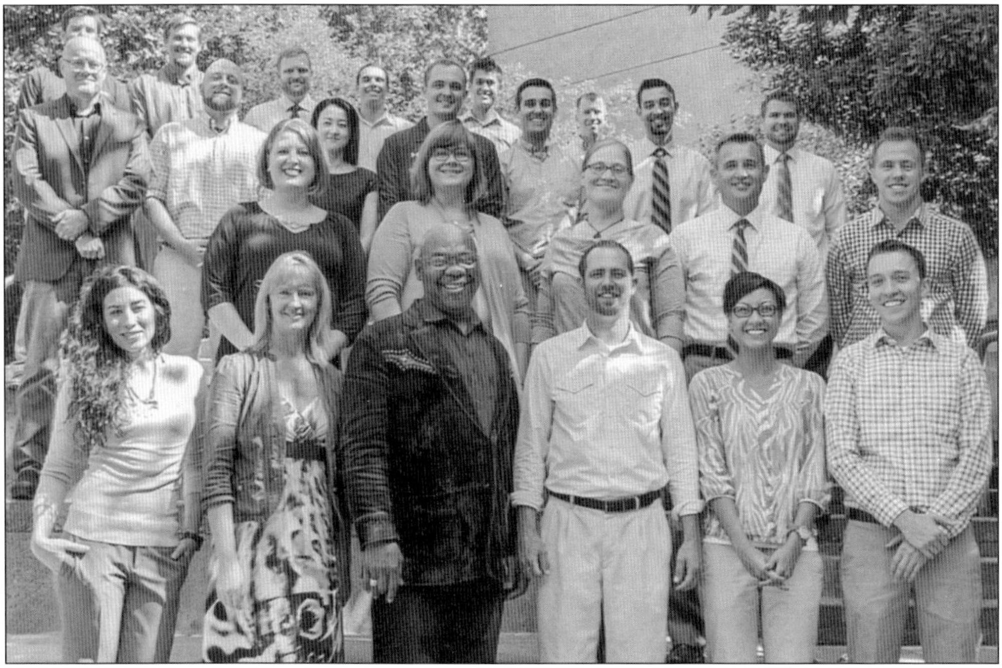

Last Yakima Class. In 2013, MEDEX decided that Class 19 would be the last Yakima class. This decision was based on a combination of issues, like the availability of clinical sites and the declining applicant pool of students from Central Washington. The last Yakima class, shown here, graduated in August 2014.

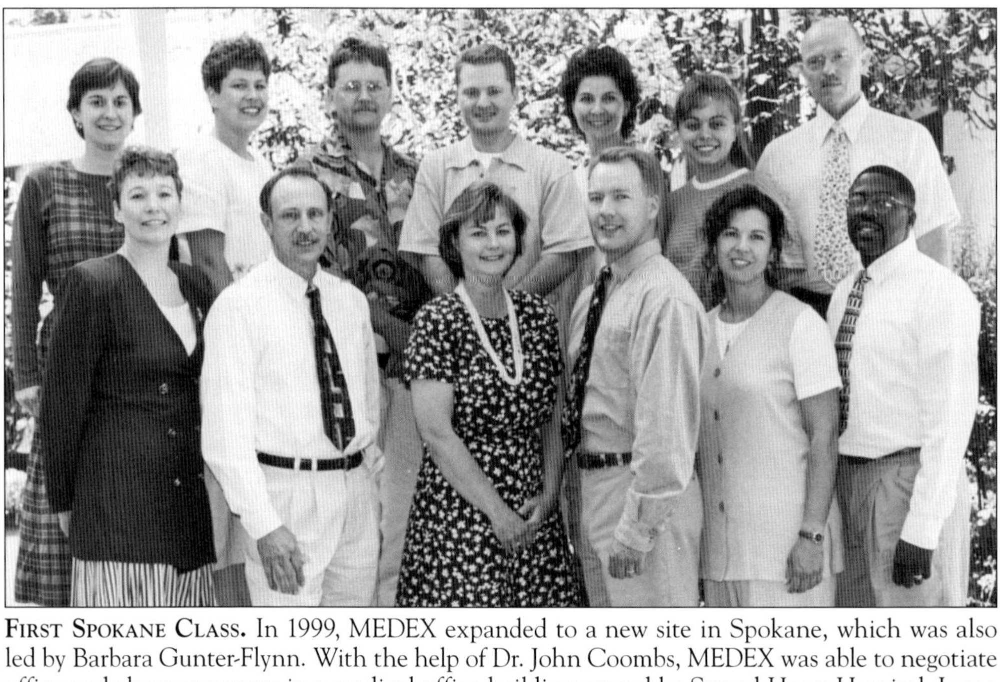

First Spokane Class. In 1999, MEDEX expanded to a new site in Spokane, which was also led by Barbara Gunter-Flynn. With the help of Dr. John Coombs, MEDEX was able to negotiate office and classroom space in a medical office building owned by Sacred Heart Hospital. Later, the classroom and then the program's offices moved onto the Eastern Washington University at Spokane Riverpoint campus.

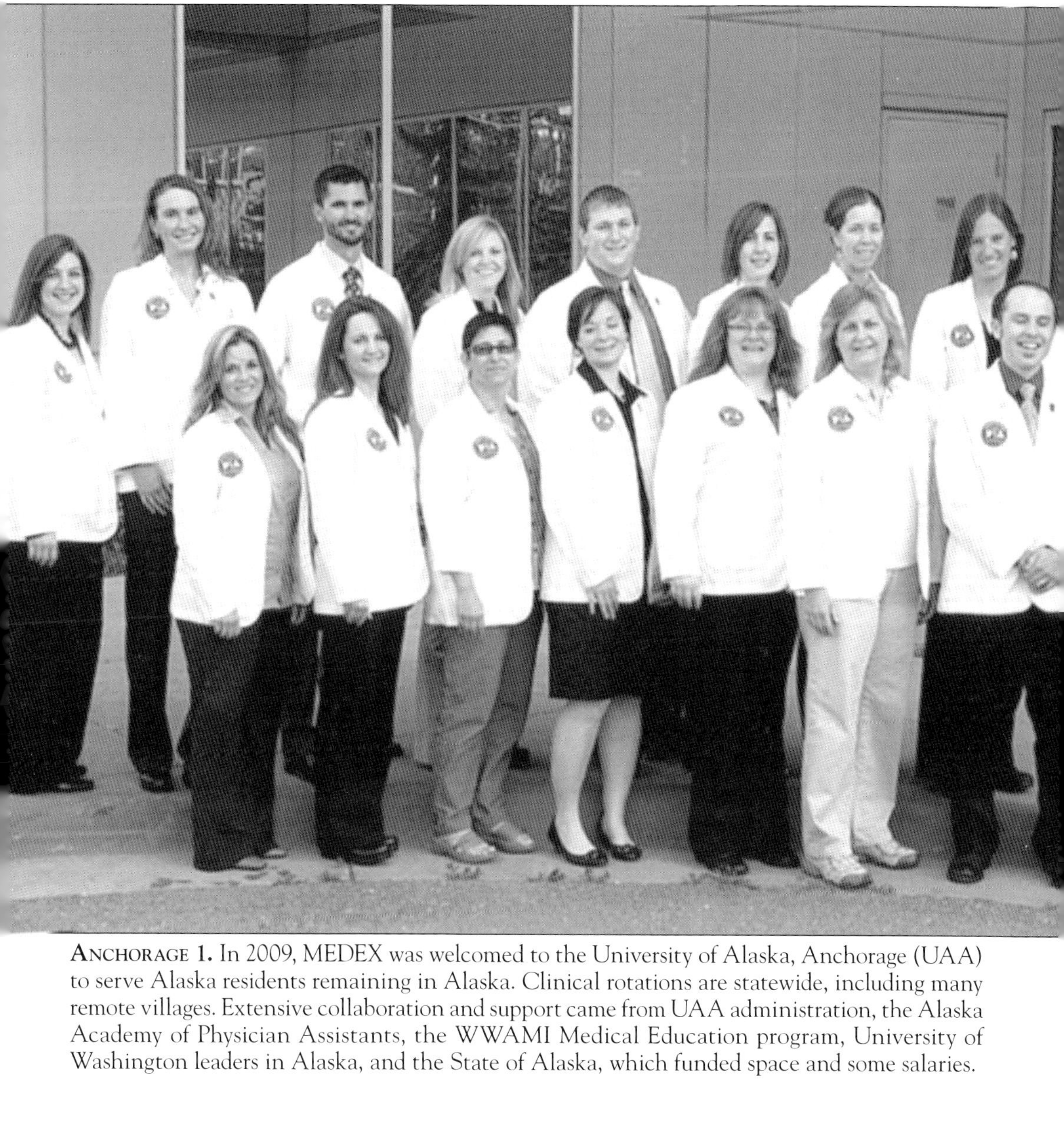

ANCHORAGE 1. In 2009, MEDEX was welcomed to the University of Alaska, Anchorage (UAA) to serve Alaska residents remaining in Alaska. Clinical rotations are statewide, including many remote villages. Extensive collaboration and support came from UAA administration, the Alaska Academy of Physician Assistants, the WWAMI Medical Education program, University of Washington leaders in Alaska, and the State of Alaska, which funded space and some salaries.

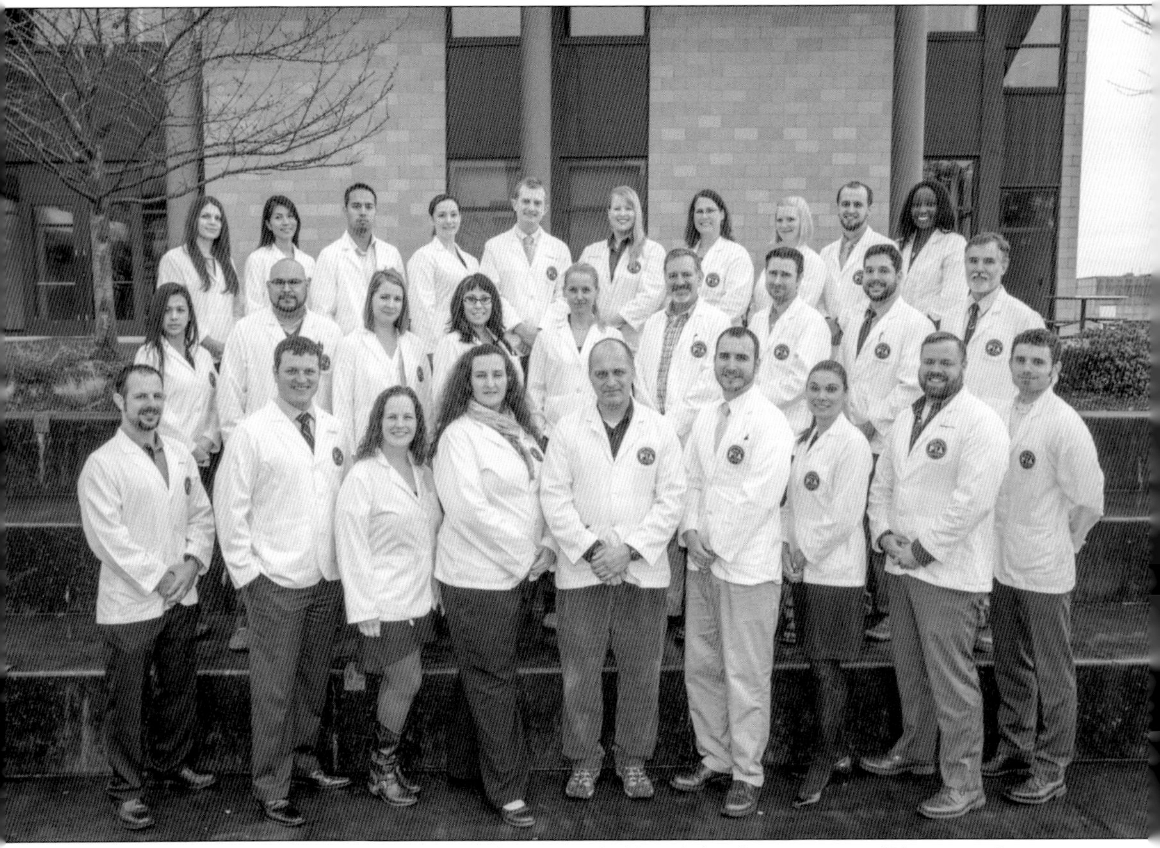

First Tacoma Class. With start-up funding provided by a federal Expansion of Physician Assistant Training (EPAT) grant, the Tacoma MEDEX site was designed to serve returning military men and women as well as students from rural communities in Southwestern Washington and the Olympic Peninsula. Chancellor Debra Friedman at the University of Washington, Tacoma, quickly integrated MEDEX into the campus with the additional support from the nursing faculty in Department of Healthcare Leadership. The first Tacoma class graduated in August 2015.

Nine

MEDEX IN ALASKA

Some of MEDEX's most important work has been done in Alaska. The extremes of geography and climate present challenges for the delivery of everything—including health care. Fortunately, MEDEX was given the opportunity to send students and develop programs in Alaska beginning with MEDEX Class 4 in the 1970s. With some federal medical support and personal linkages and friendships developed through the Peace Corps, MEDEX sent seven Class 4 students to Alaska based on decisions made by interviewers and MEDEX staff at their admissions interviews. These seven students completed their clinical training in Alaska and remained to demonstrate the PA career's possibilities in many settings throughout the state. This first cohort of Alaska PAs, and those who quickly followed them, were all former military corpsmen.

They were quickly accepted in Alaska settings, including remote villages and small towns, and laid a strong foundation for the new career as they worked diligently to create Alaska's PA regulatory process. Joe Marzucco (Class 4), wrote about this experience in the *Journal of the American Academy of Physician Assistants.*

The PA career gained national visibility when PAs became the medical providers during the building of the Alaska pipeline. Under the guidance of Dr. Philip Nice, a group of PAs with occupational medicine and trauma skills rotated in and out of the pipeline pumping stations and became an integral part of the pipeline legend.

MEDEX began formally admitting Alaskans, including Alaska community health aides, into the MEDEX program in 1981. New roles were created including teaching and supervising health aides for the native corporations. In 1993, MEDEX opened its first Alaska training site in Sitka; however, a dramatic decrease in oil revenues resulted in its closure after the graduation of its first class. In 2000, a new MEDEX training site opened in Anchorage in partnership with the University of Alaska. Alaska remains the state with the most PAs per capita in the nation.

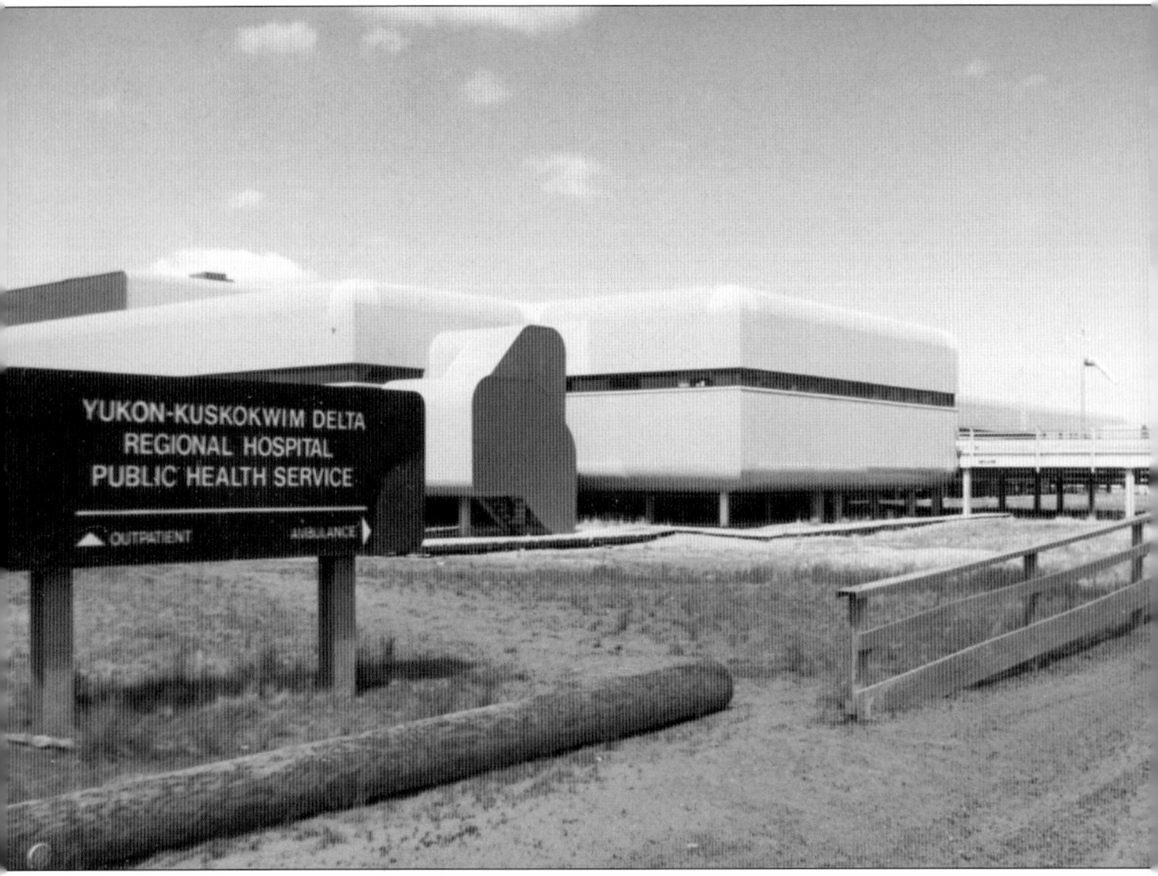

Off the Road System. The Yukon-Kuskokwim Health Corporation (YKHC) operates this hospital for Bethel, Alaska, approximately 400 miles west of Anchorage, with access only by air and river. YKHC also operates clinics for five subregional areas, and clinics for 56 villages staffed by community health aides. Many MEDEX students have trained with the YKHC, which employs PAs as clinicians, health worker trainers, and village health supervisors. (Author's collection.)

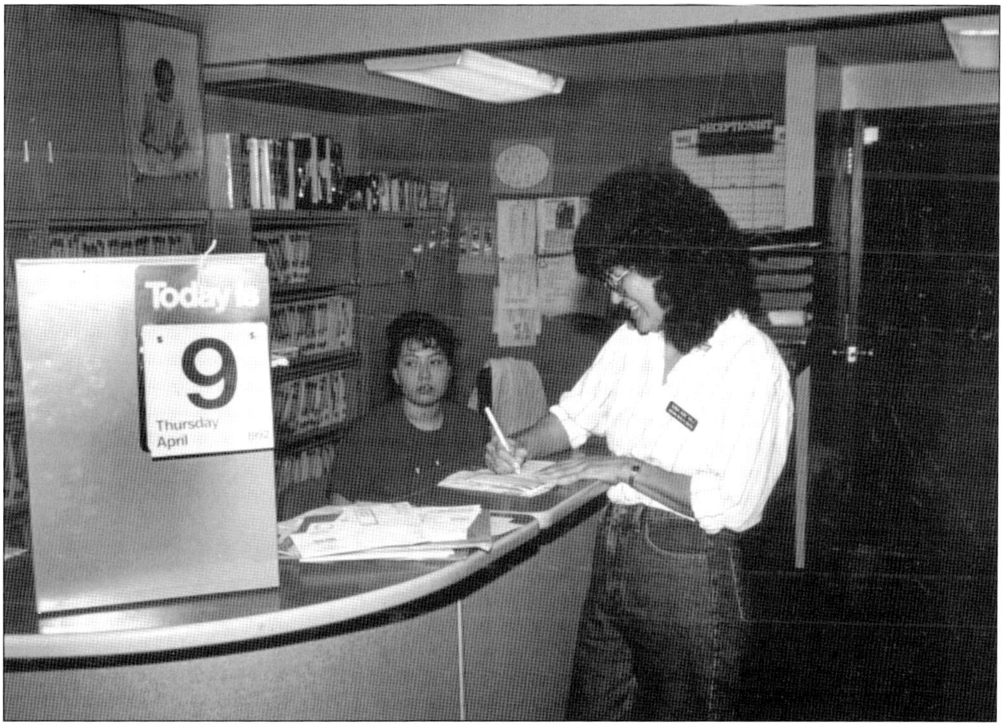

COMMUNITY HEALTH AIDES TRAINED AS PAs. Sonia Vent (Class 17) is one of many Alaskans who entered MEDEX with a strong clinical background as a community health aide. She is seen here in a village clinic.

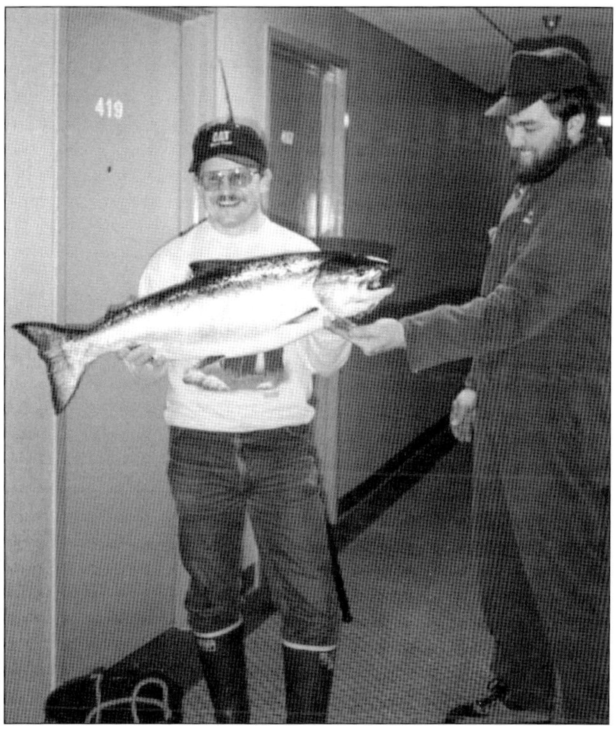

PRINCE OF WALES ISLAND. Kurt Welser (Sitka Class) was a nurse and EMT on Prince of Wales Island in Southeast Alaska prior to becoming a PA in the Sitka MEDEX class. He is shown at left with Sitka classmate Larry Fisher. Welser helped the City of Thorne Bay start a medical clinic in 1982. He worked for the Southeast Alaska Regional Health Corporation (SEARHC) in rural clinics in Kake, Klawock, and Hydaburg. (Courtesy of Kurt Welser.)

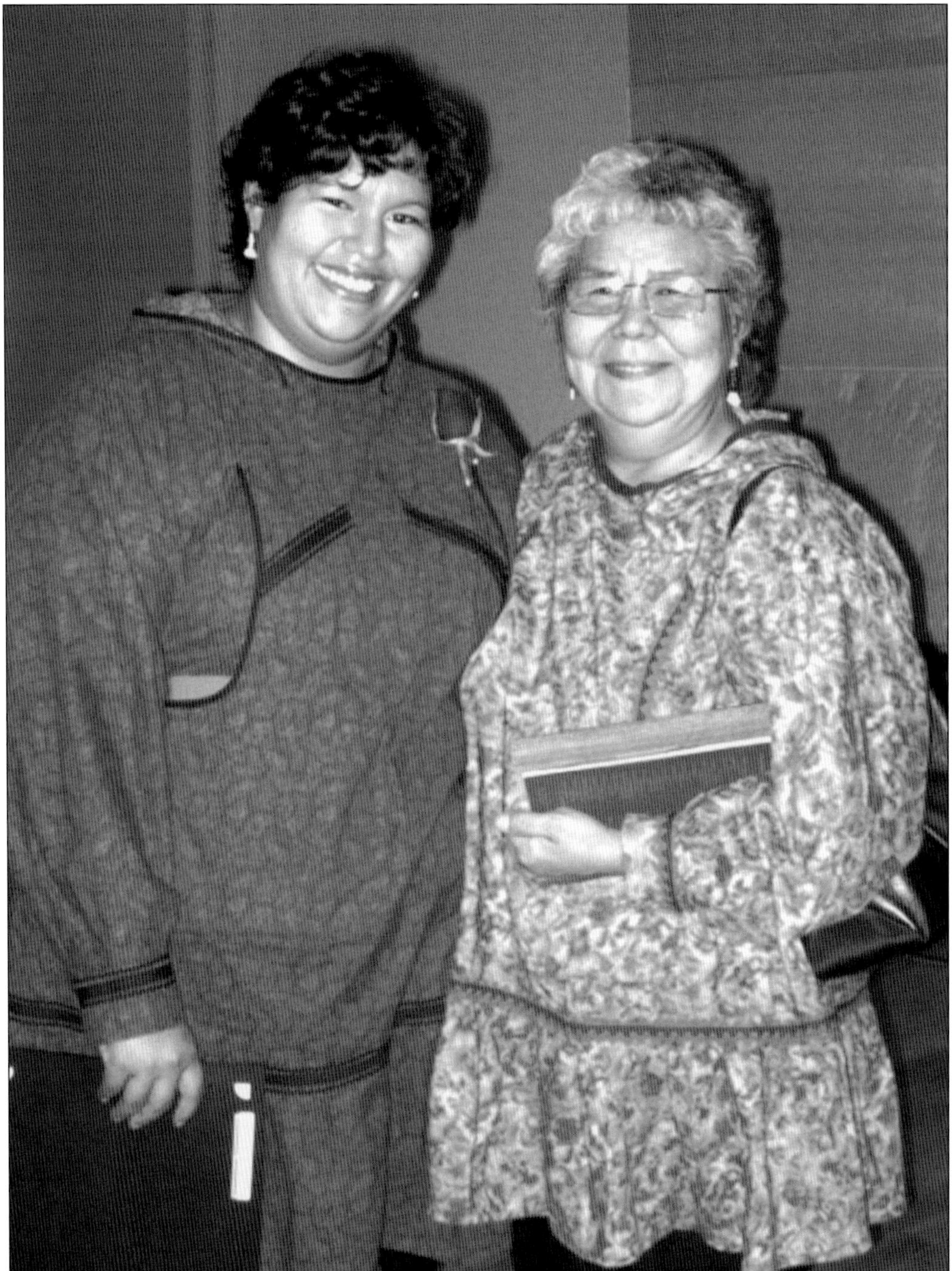

Two Generations. Martha Flores (Seattle 23, right) was a health aide in Mountain Home, Alaska, prior to coming to MEDEX. Martha's daughter Teresa (Seattle 37, left) also became a PA at MEDEX. The two are shown at Teresa's graduation. Martha's career has been spent in emergency medicine and primary care in Bethel, Alaska, with the Yukon Kuskokwim Health Corporation (YKHC); Teresa also worked at YKHC and has also served on the MEDEX faculties in both Seattle and Anchorage.

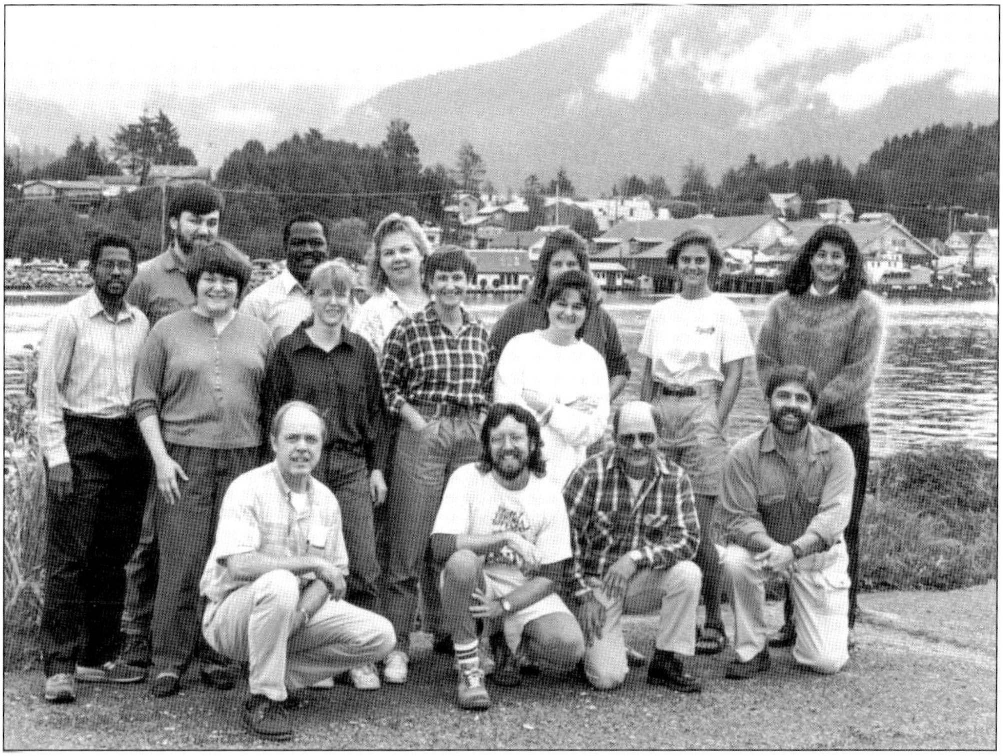

SITKA CLASS PORTRAIT. Now out of the elevator (see page 98) and into the field, the Sitka class poses with faculty member Grace Landel (third row, far right). In its short-term impact from 1993–1994, the innovative program helped to launch the reputation of the PA profession in the state, paving the way for the Anchorage satellite to open in 2009.

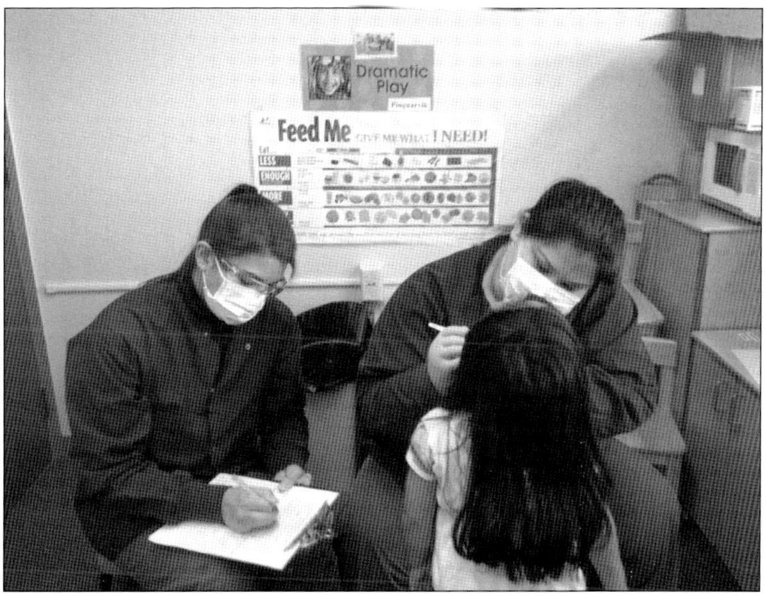

HOLISTIC CARE. DENTEX students team up on a child exam. The wall poster shows brightly colored food alternatives and options. The decorative conversation piece reflects clinical encouragement for healthy choices and affirms nutritious traditional local foods.

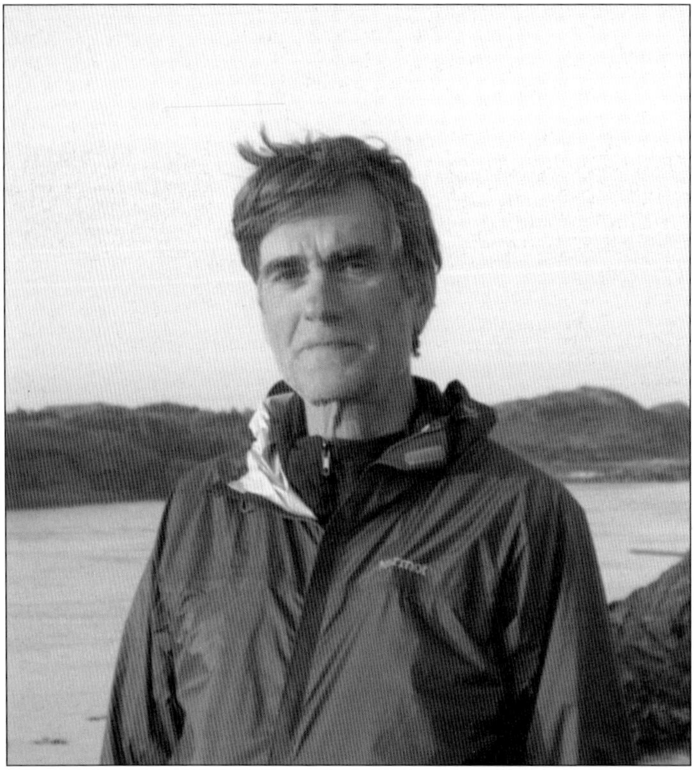

ANCHORAGE FACULTY LEADER. John Riley is a graduate of the PA program at the University of Wisconsin. He has worked for many years in Alaska and still continues to provide primary care at the Anchorage Neighborhood Health Center. With an additional background in public health, Riley first served as the Alaska clinical coordinator for MEDEX based at the University of Alaska. He was instrumental in the development of the Alaska MEDEX site and served as the leader of the site until his retirement in 2015. (Courtesy of John Riley.)

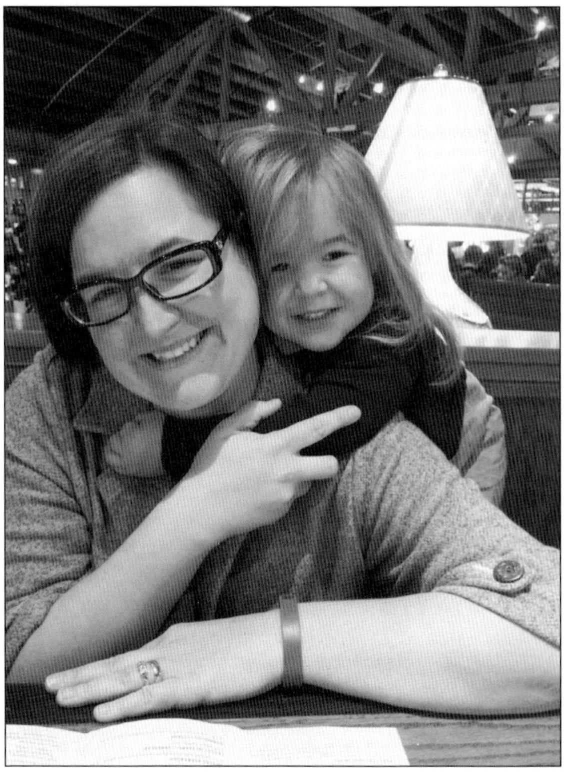

FOUNDING ALASKA FACULTY MEMBER. Denise Coslett completed a masters in PA studies at King's College, Pennsylvania, and moved to Anchorage to work for the Indian Health Service and the South Central Foundation as an emergency room PA. Coslett was a founding member of the Anchorage site, teaching emergency medicine, adult medicine, and other topics. Now the PA leader in the emergency room at the Alaska Native Medical Center, Coslett also teaches in the DENTEX dental therapy program. She is pictured here with her daughter Bryn. (Courtesy of Denise Coslett.)

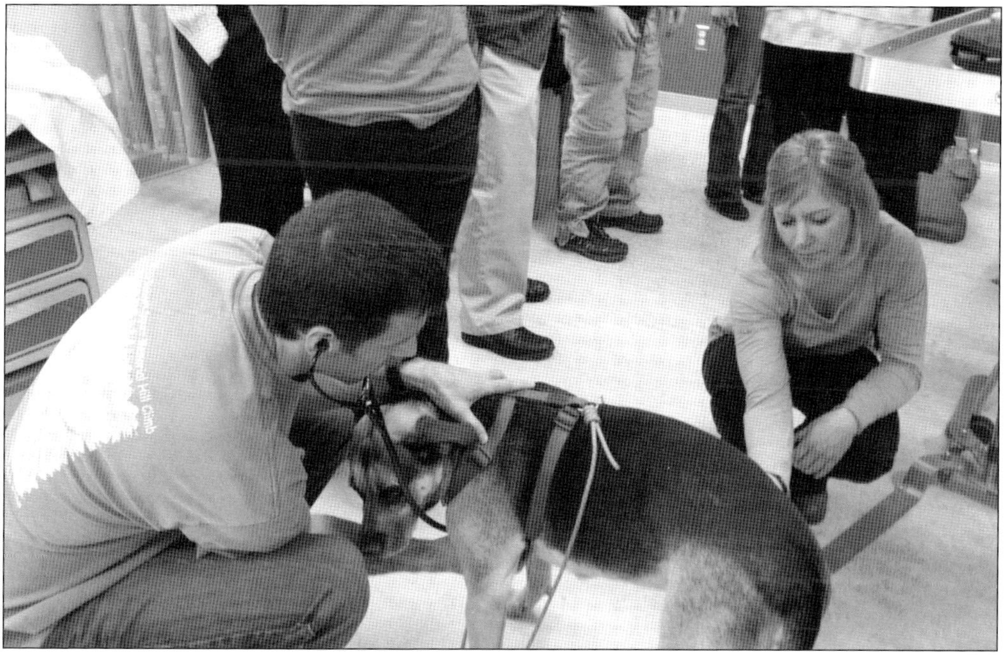

Students Learn Veterinary Skills. A unique feature of PA practice in remote Alaska villages is treating precious dogs when veterinary care is not available. The MEDEX Alaska faculty arranged unique dog veterinary workshops. Students and their "patients" are pictured here. (Courtesy of Pat Hensch.)

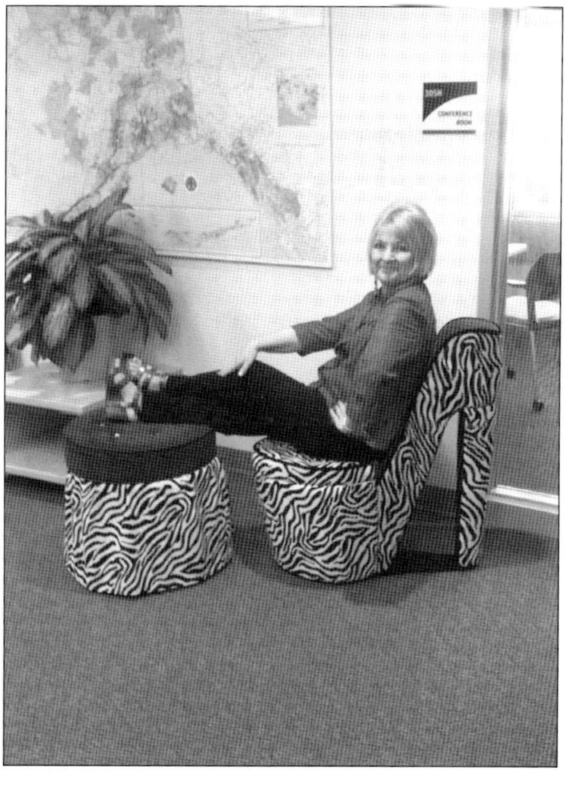

Alaska Clinical Coordinator. Pat Hensch (Class 19) served as clinical coordinator for the Alaska MEDEX site. Originally from Minnesota, she lived in Bethel, Alaska, when she became a MEDEX student in Seattle. She later worked in many capacities, including correctional health, health aide training, and primary care. As clinical coordinator, Hensch traveled throughout Alaska to develop clinical training sites and to evaluate students in small, rural, and remote communities.

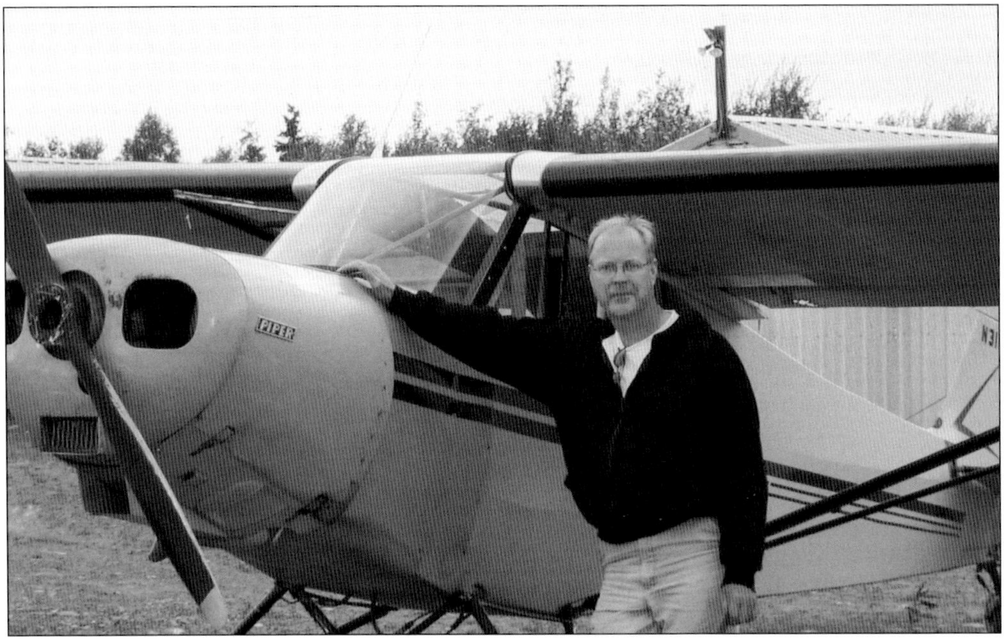

Faculty PA and Pilot. Ashley Marquardt (Class 33) is an Air Force veteran with extensive primary-care and emergency-medicine clinical experience throughout Alaska, including in villages and urban Anchorage. As a man who "lives to fly and also to play hockey," Marquardt is pictured with one of his Piper Cubs at a small airport near Anchorage. (Courtesy of Ashley Marquardt.)

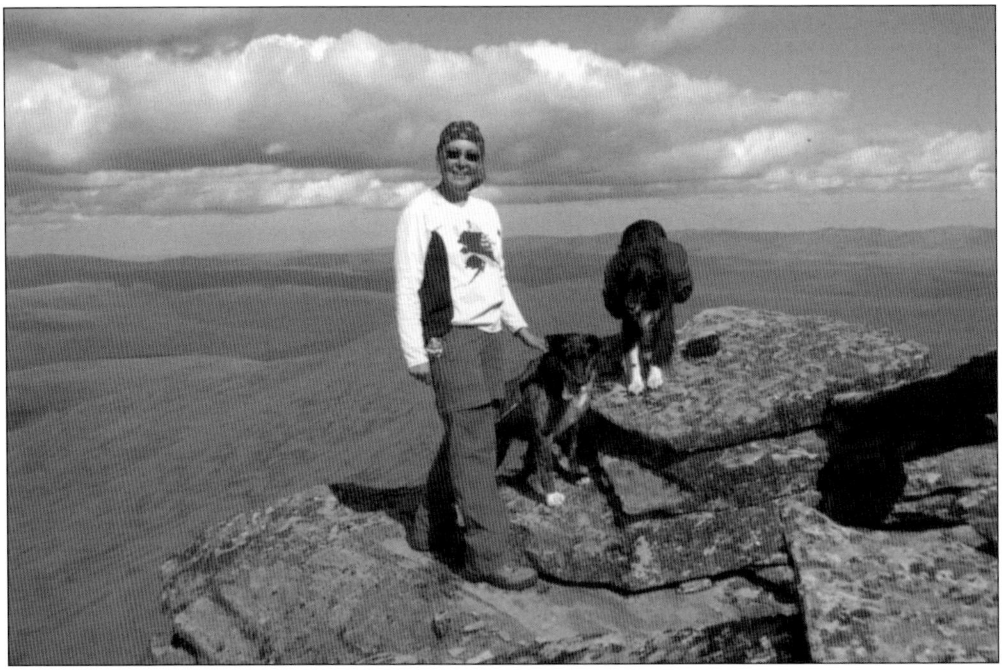

PA Faculty Adventurer. Robin Cope (Class 38) has extensive experience in emergency medicine. She joined the Anchorage faculty in 2013 in a variety of roles including lecturer, advisor, and clinical coordinator. Cope's hobbies focus on the outdoors. She is shown here backpacking with her two dogs on a Pinnell Mountain trail north of Fairbanks. (Courtesy of Robin Cope.)

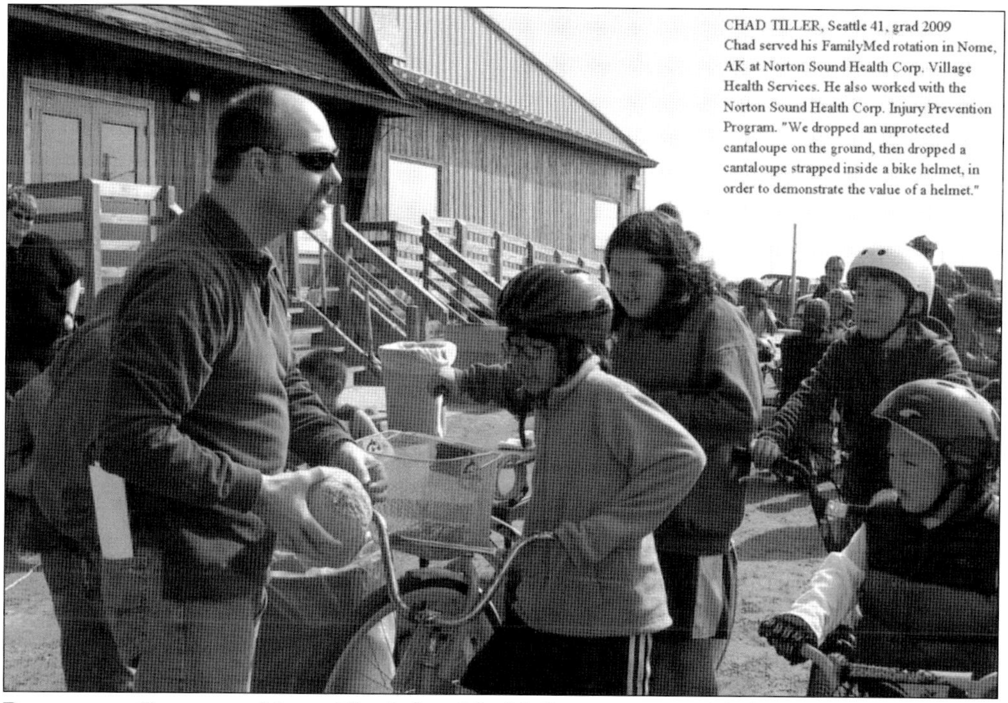

CHAD TILLER, Seattle 41, grad 2009
Chad served his FamilyMed rotation in Nome, AK at Norton Sound Health Corp. Village Health Services. He also worked with the Norton Sound Health Corp. Injury Prevention Program. "We dropped an unprotected cantaloupe on the ground, then dropped a cantaloupe strapped inside a bike helmet, in order to demonstrate the value of a helmet."

Prevention Project in Nome. The Indian Health Service Hospital, led by Dr. David Head, has been an outstanding primary-care preceptorship site for MEDEX students. Here in Nome, Chad Tiller (Class 41) has organized a community outreach event promoting the use of bicycle helmets. In this demonstration, he drops one cantaloupe wearing a bicycle helmet and one cantaloupe without one to compare the results to his concerned young audience. (Courtesy of Chad Tiller.)

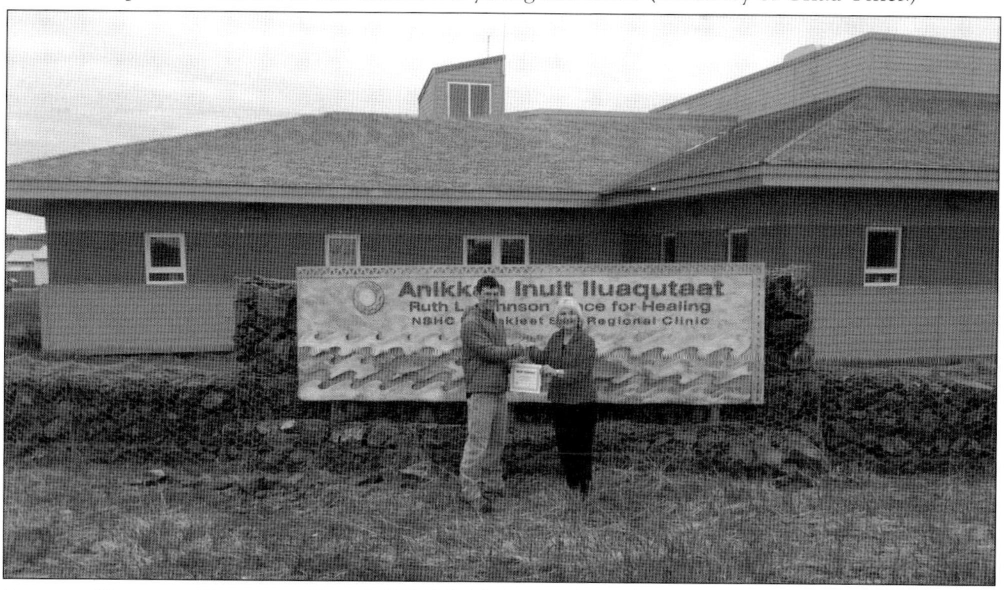

Remote Clinical Training Site. MEDEX Alaska students have been successful in applying for external scholarships to support their training. Here, Pat Hensch is seen presenting a scholarship from the AAPA Veterans Caucus to Nathan Greene during his rotation at Anikkan Inuit Iluaqutaat Unalakleet Clinic.

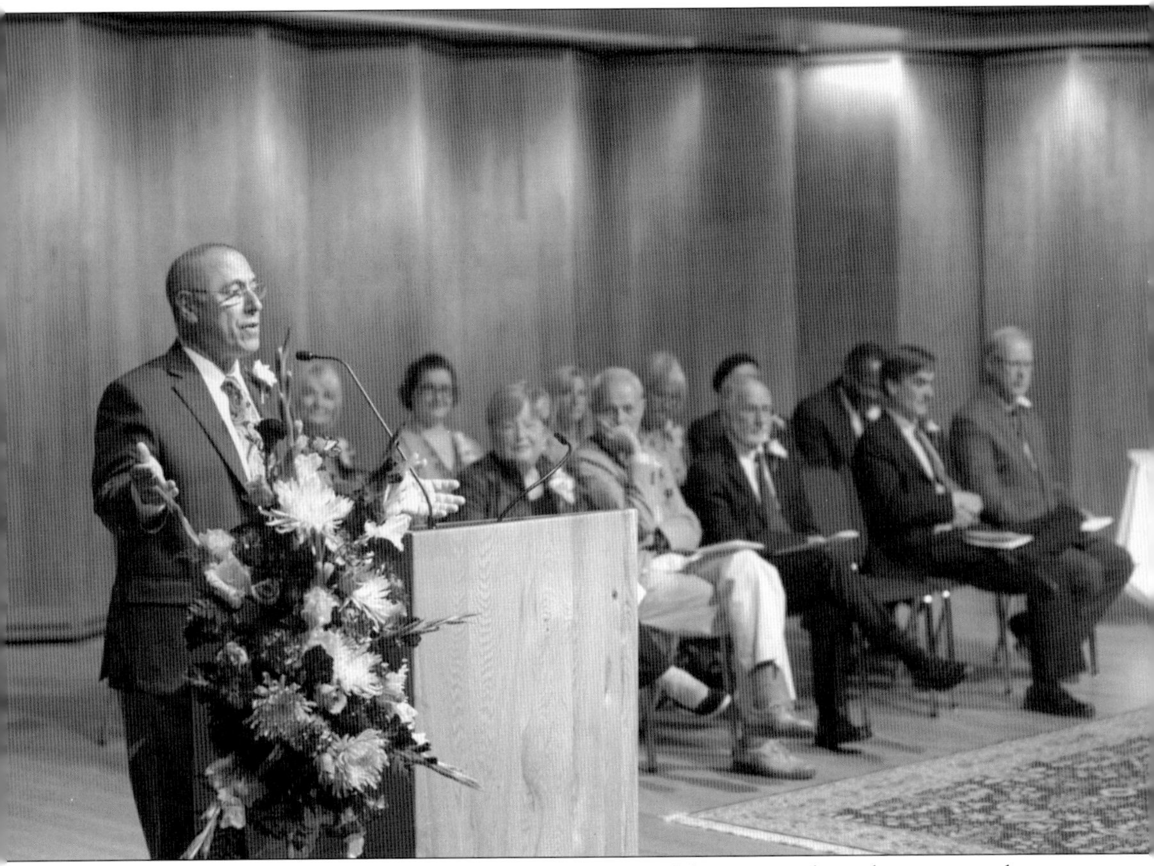

Class 4 Graduates. Joseph Marzucco (Class 4) was one of the seven early graduates sent to become Alaska's first PAs. Pictured here at the podium, he addresses the Anchorage Class 4 graduates in 2014. Seated from left to right are (first row) Ruth Ballweg; Dr. Thomas Nighswander, WWAMI Alaska dean for clinical affairs; William Hogan, dean of the UAA School of Health Professions; John Riley, Alaska site director; and Ashley Marquardt, Alaska faculty member; (second row) Alaska faculty members Pat Hensch and Denise Coslett; Sara Bigelow, president of the Alaska Academy of Physician Assistants; Robin Cope, Anchorage faculty member; Gino Gianola, Seattle faculty member; and Terry Scott, program director.

Ten

INTERNATIONAL ACTIVITIES AND THE FUTURE

The growth and expanded use of PAs in the United States has gained increased visibility internationally. MEDEX graduates have facilitated and personify this growth. Serving as PAs in all four branches of the US military, the US Department of State, the Peace Corps, and the US Public Health Service, MEDEX graduates have been visible ambassadors for the PA profession. Similarly, MEDEX PAs employed by global corporations, nongovernmental organizations, and religious service projects have extended the hands of care to those without access due to geography, resources, or discrimination. They have also made themselves quickly available to respond to disasters and epidemics including the September 11, 2001, terrorist attacks, the Indonesian tsunami, Hurricane Katrina in New Orleans, and the disease outbreaks that followed the earthquake in Haiti.

As other countries have contemplated adapting the US physician assistant model to their specific needs, PAs from MEDEX have joined pilot projects designed to introduce PAs into these countries' health-care workforces. The United Kingdom's first pilot focused on primary care. The pilot for Queensland, Australia, was designed with a special concern for health-care access in remote communities. South Australia piloted PAs in surgical roles. Health Workforce New Zealand piloted generalist roles in small communities. MEDEX PAs were competitively chosen for all of these pilots. Their pictures are included in this chapter.

Simultaneously, the MEDEX program itself has welcomed clinicians, policy makers, and faculty from other countries to share Dick Smith's principles and the program's experience in creating and developing the PA profession globally. Visitors have included representatives from Ghana, South Africa, three provinces in Canada, Australia, New Zealand, China, the United Kingdom, Mozambique, and Guyana. MEDEX faculty members have provided consultation to five universities in Canada, three universities in Australia, two medical schools in New Zealand, one medical school in Ireland, two programs in Ghana, and three programs in South Africa.

In addition, MEDEX has digitized the 35 volumes of the MEDEX Primary Care Series, and plans further editing and expansion of the content for electronic distribution to health worker programs globally.

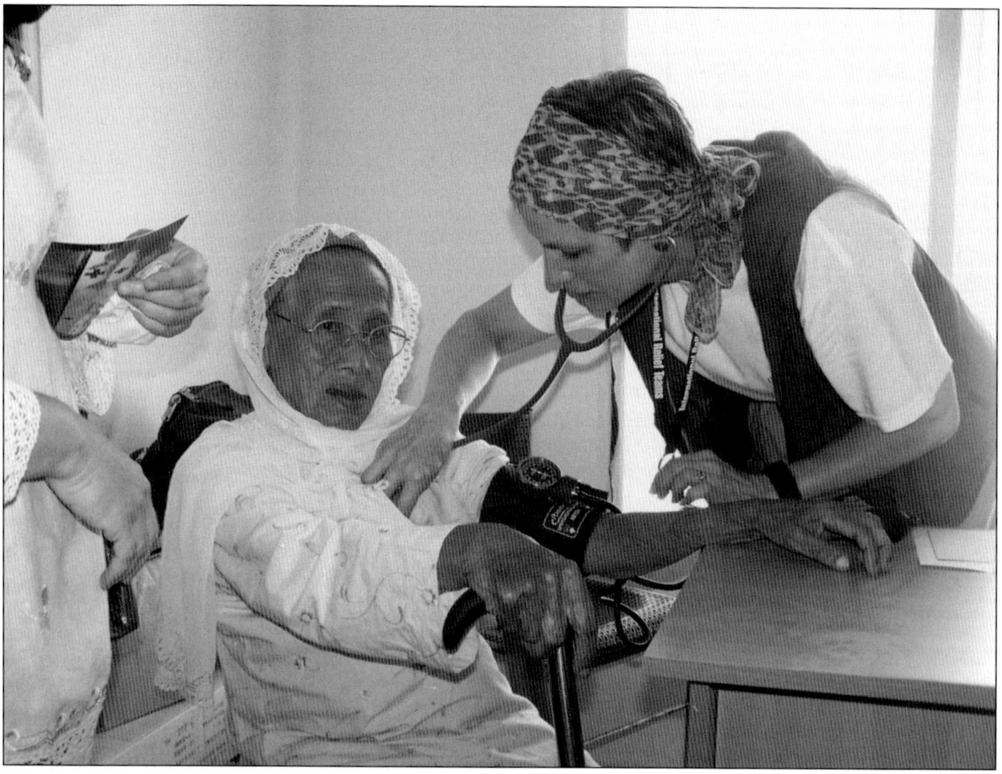

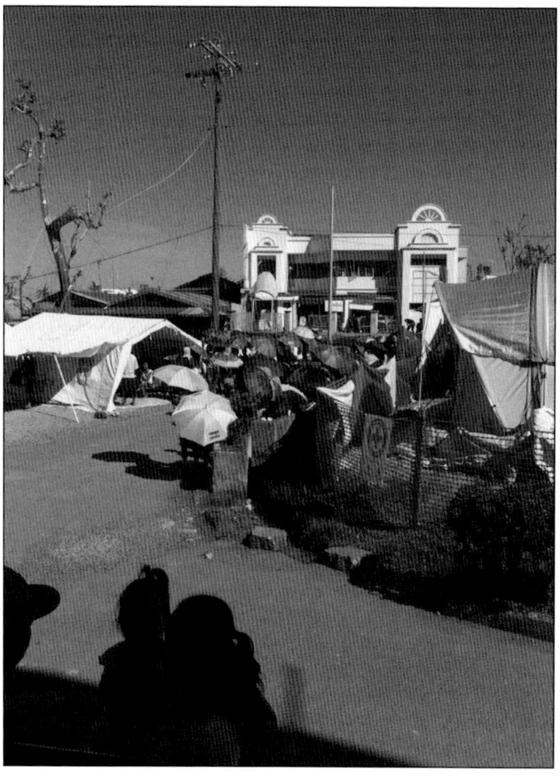

Resilience Abroad. Nanette Laufik (Class 19) cares for a woman in Indonesia on a humanitarian assistance deployment with the USNS *Mercy*, one of two hospital ships for the US Navy. Laufik has volunteered her time as a PA under crisis conditions in countries including Afghanistan and Albania.

Typhoon Recovery. This tent clinic in the Philippines was set up for survivors of Typhoon Haiyan in November 2013. The storm, with winds up to 196 miles per hour, caused a loss of over 6,300 lives in the Philippines alone. Larry Applebee (Yakima 8) provided this photograph of operations from his volunteer work as a PA in disaster recovery.

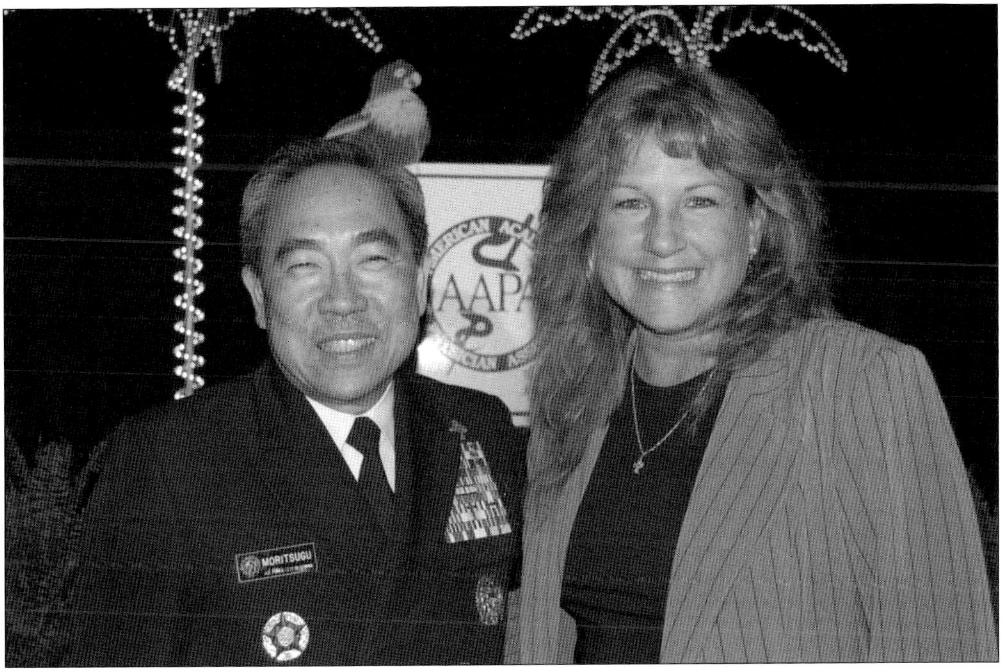

AAPA IN 2007. Laurie Benton (Class 26) has served as a volunteer PA after Hurricane Katrina and in other emergency-care settings. Here, she converses with Rear Admiral Dr. Kenneth Moritsugu, MD, former US surgeon general. (Courtesy of Laurie Benton.)

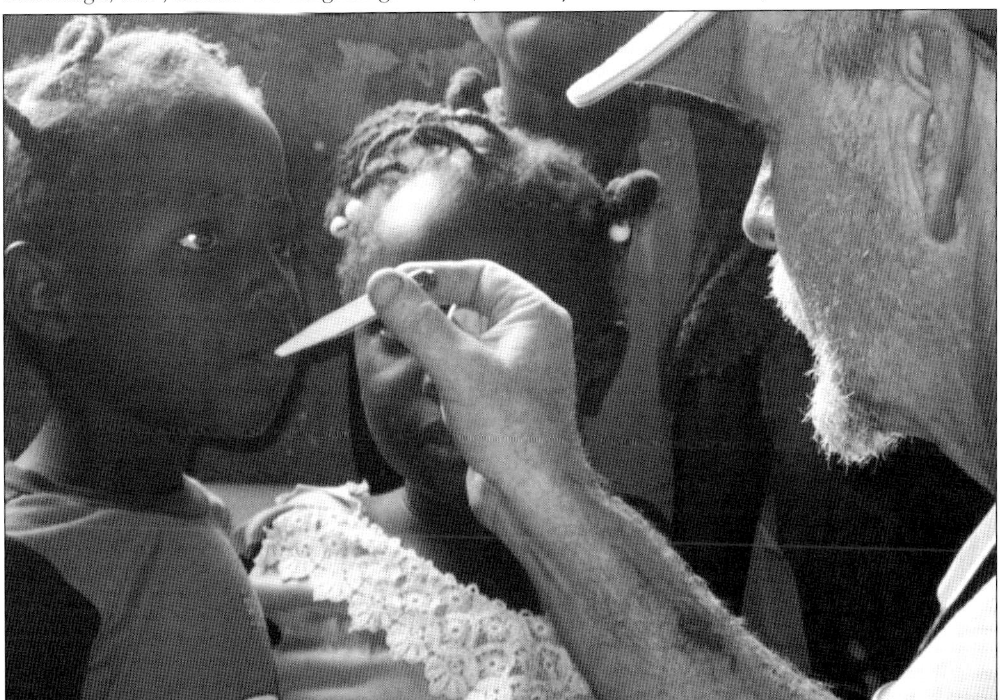

HAITI RESPONSE. Larry Applebee (Yakima 8) is shown working in Haiti after the earthquake. (Courtesy of Larry Applebee.)

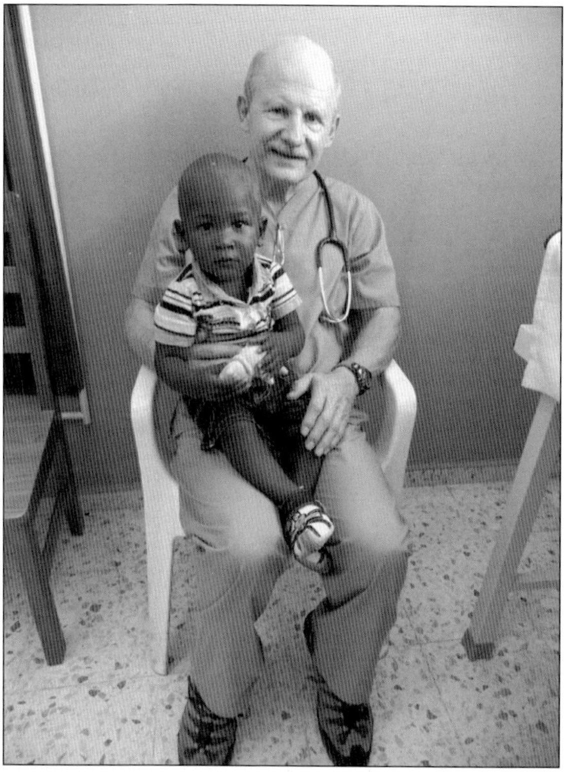

Alaska Volunteer. Kurt Welser (Sitka Class) is shown here as a medical volunteer in the Dominican Republic. (Courtesy of Kurt Welser.)

PAs in Cambodia. MEDEX graduates from three different classes worked together in 2012 with Vets with a Mission providing medical care to villages around Siem Reap, Cambodia, and on the floating villages on the Vietnam-Cambodia border. From left to right are Fred Belau (Class 3), Nhumey Tropp (Class 14), and Robin Moore (Class 35). (Courtesy of Robin Moore.)

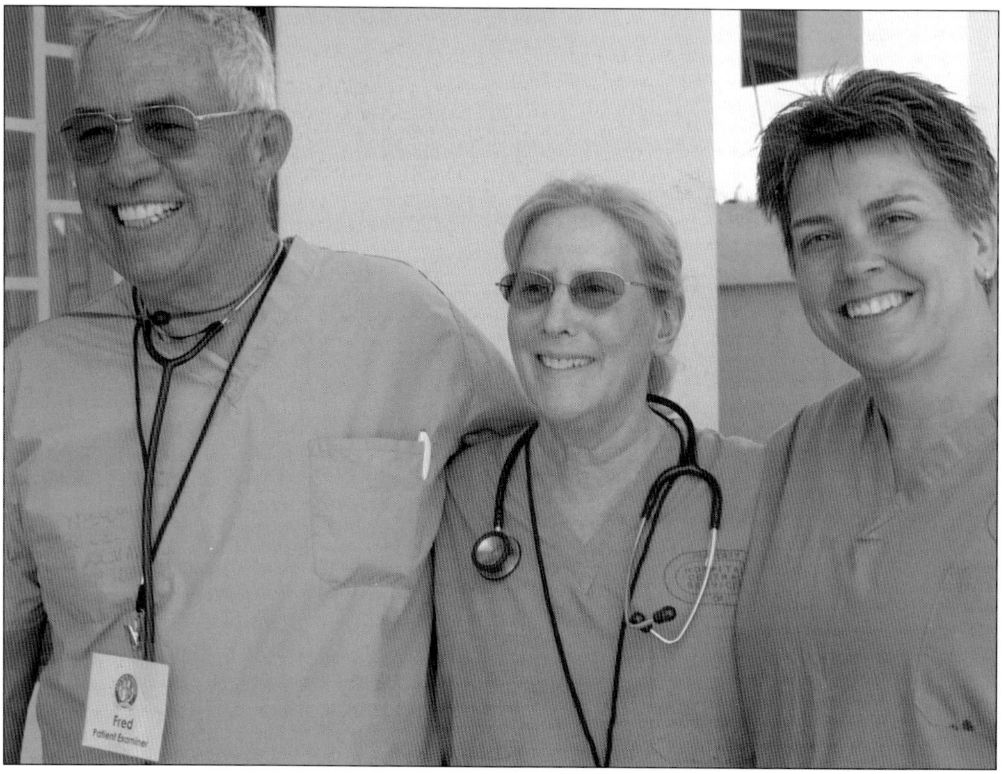

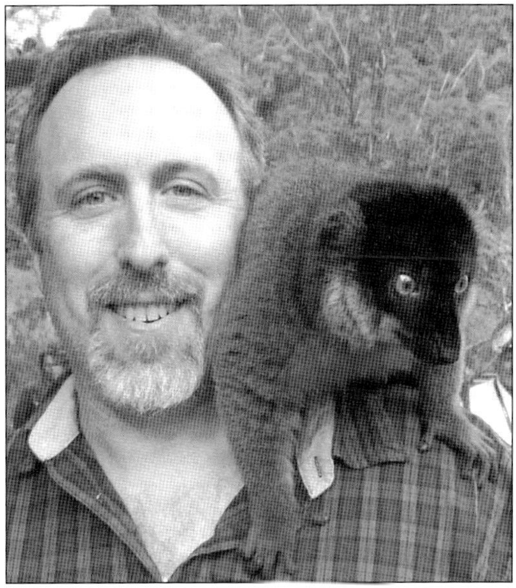

Madagascar. Chris Carson has worked internationally throughout his career. He says, "Working for the US Department of State in embassies around the world, we are our diplomat's primary providers and become our own family providers. I personally know of three MEDEX graduates doing the same thing." In a nonclinical picture, Carson is shown with a lemur in Madagascar. (Courtesy of Chris Carson.)

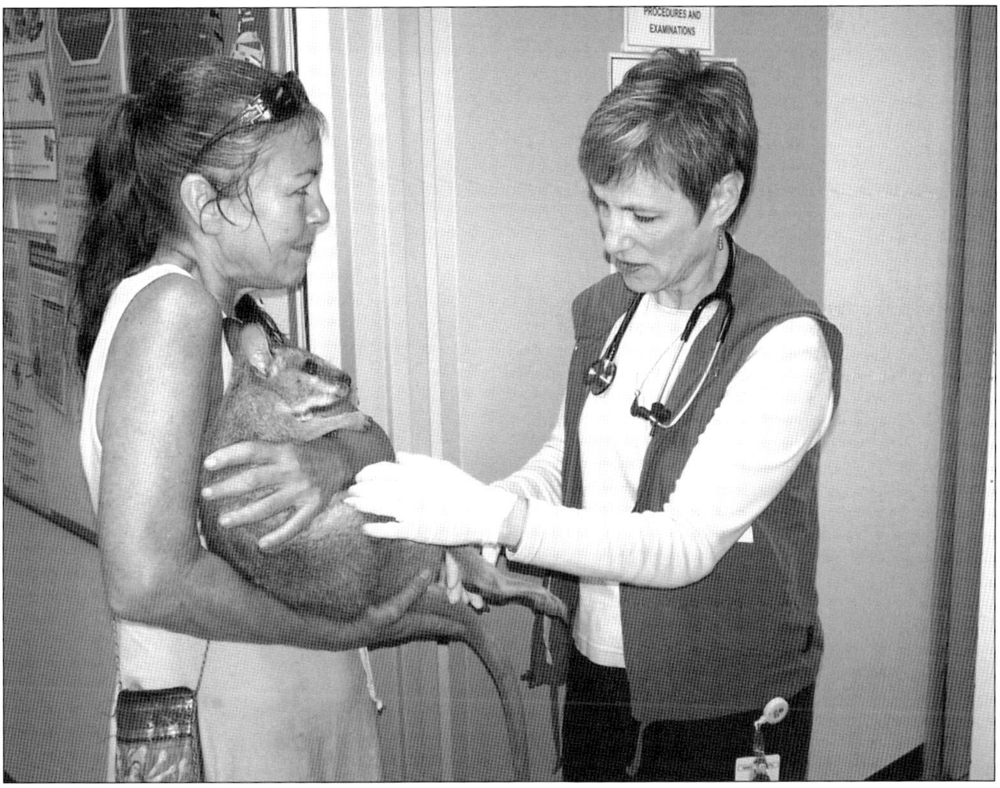

Wallaby Patient. In remote communities, PAs might care for animals as well as people. Nanette Laufik (Class 19) examines a wallaby in Cooktown, Queensland. Laufik, along with Sarah Leet (Class 31) and Elona Turk (Class 22), were three MEDEX graduates who served in the Queensland Ministry of Health pilot. Laufik and Leet worked in the historic coastal aboriginal community of Cooktown. Turk worked in the Outback mining community of Mount Isa. (Courtesy of Nanette Laufik.)

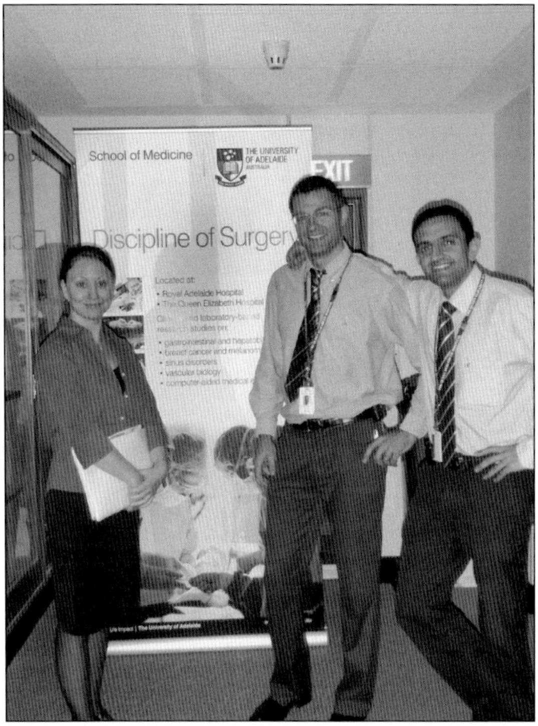

Adelaide Surgical Practice. Dawanda Pesicka (Class 35, left) stands with two surgical colleagues in the Department of Surgery at the School of Medicine, University of Adelaide, South Australia. Pesicka worked in the surgical PA pilot in Adelaide.

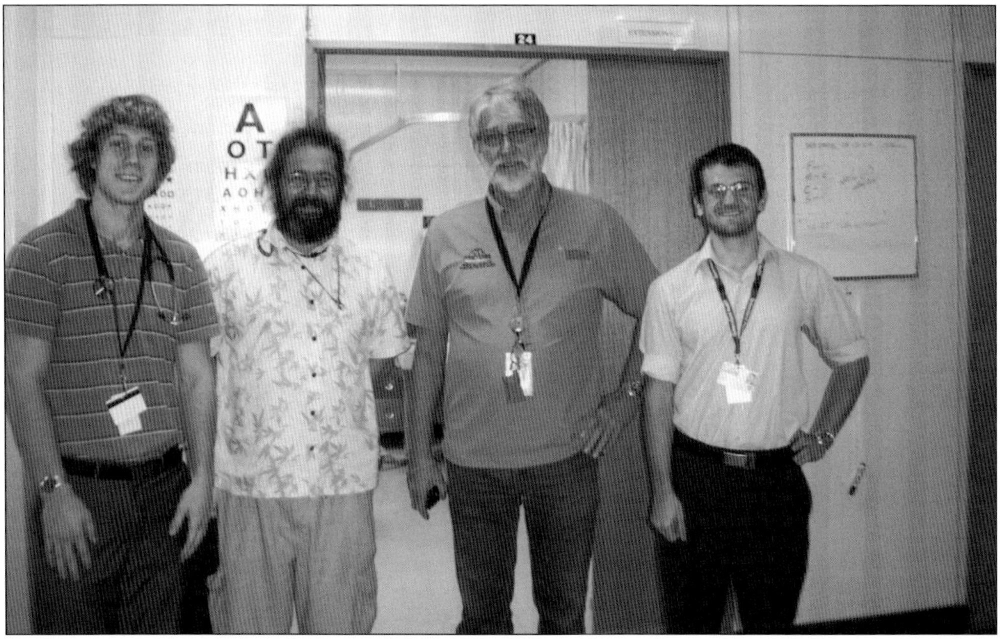

Remote Doctors. Australian doctors in small communities have been major supporters of the PA movement in Australia. The Australia College of Rural and Remote Medicine (ACRRM) provides additional training, credentialing, and support for doctors in isolated communities. Here, Dr. Dennis Pashen (second from right) is shown with young rural doctors in a hospital on the Atherton Tablelands. As the president of ACRRM, Pashen has been a strong leader, sponsor, and spokesperson for PAs in Australia. (Author's collection.)

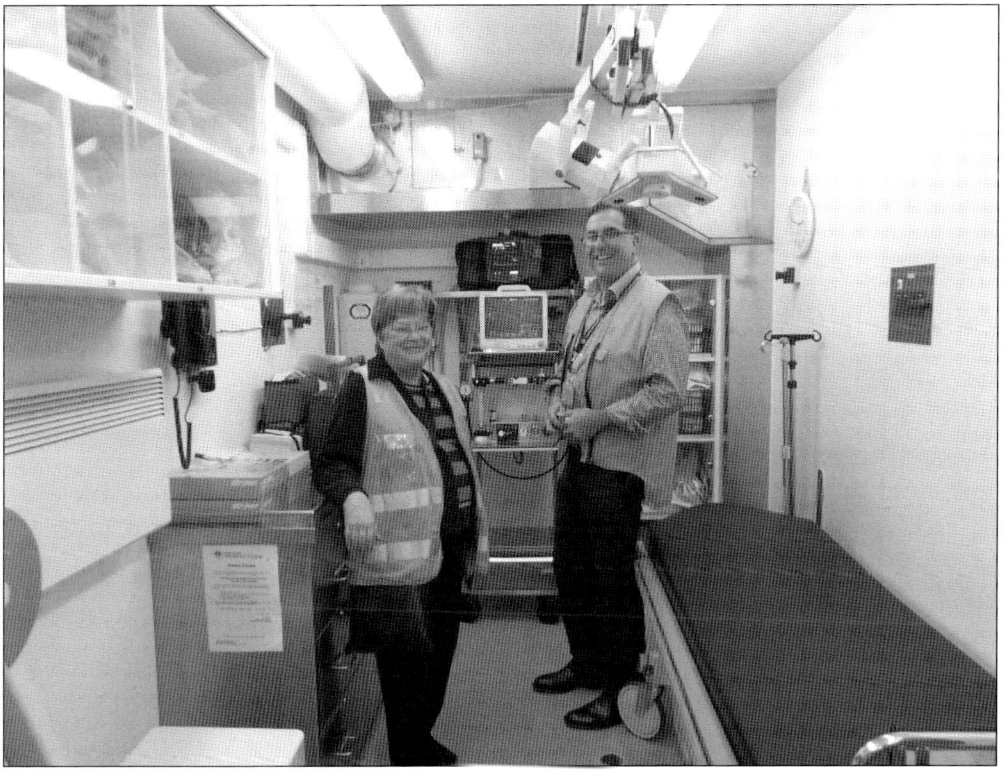

Australia Antarctica Project. While Australia does not utilize PAs to staff its four Antarctica research stations, Dr. Jeffrey Ayton leads the medical operations for the Australian Antarctic Division. He is also a past president of ACCRM. In December 2014, Ruth Ballweg visited Dr. Ayton, who demonstrated the division's compact and adaptable mobile operating room in a shipping container. (Author's collection.)

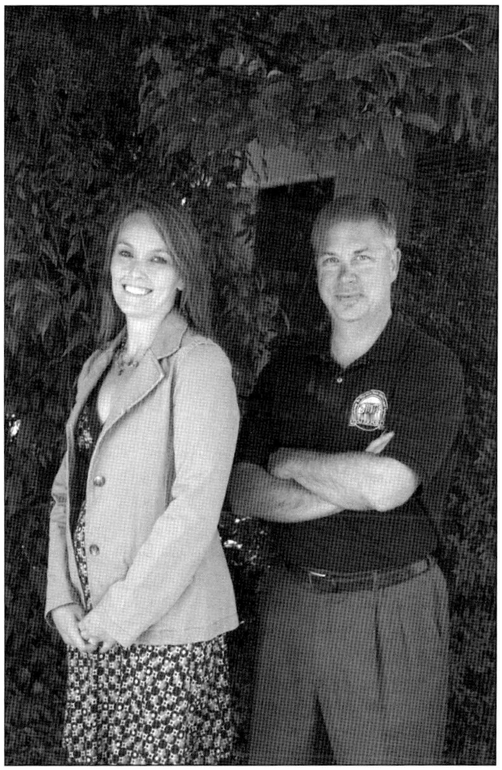

Tacoma to the United Kingdom. Founding Tacoma faculty members Vanessa Bester (left) and Drew Garcia are shown at the Tacoma site. Garcia has accepted a faculty position with the new United Kingdom PA program at the University of Worcester.

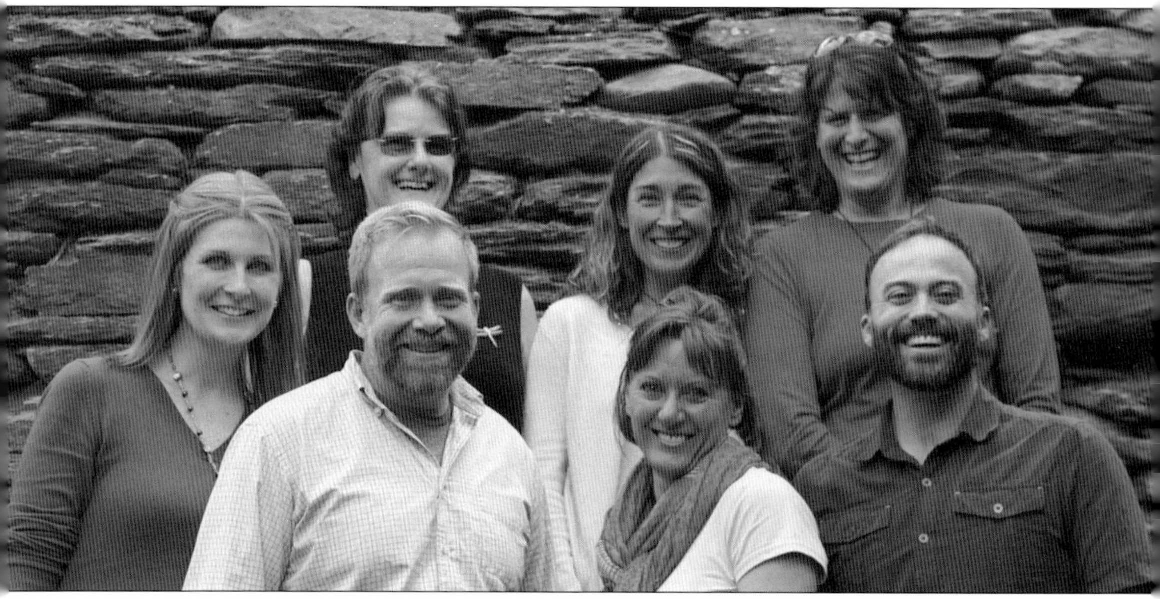

PAs in New Zealand. Seven PAs, five of them MEDEX graduates, were chosen to participate in the two-year PA pilot sponsored by the New Zealand Ministry of Health. The group agreed to follow the path of PAs in the United Kingdom and adopt the title "physician associate." They worked together to create and formalize the New Zealand Academy of Physician Assistants. From left to right are (first row) George Froehle (Class 40), Machelle Dotson (Spokane 10), and Jeremy Palmer (Class 41); (second row) Tiffany Hodgson, Gail Tharpe-Lucero (Spokane 6), Amee Koch (Yakima 7), and Lis Gammelin. (Courtesy of Machelle Dotson.)

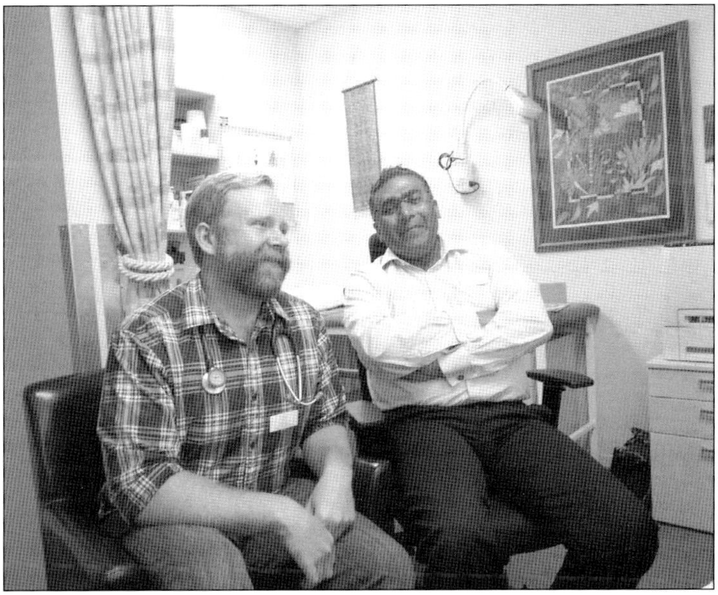

New Zealand Preceptor. George Froehle (Class 40, left) worked in a primary-care clinic owned by Radius Inc. in Hamilton, New Zealand, with his supervising doctor, Dr. Stanley Koshi (right). As one of the last US physician assistants to leave the New Zealand pilot program, Froehle has continued to work on PA regulation with the New Zealand Medical Association. (Author's collection.)

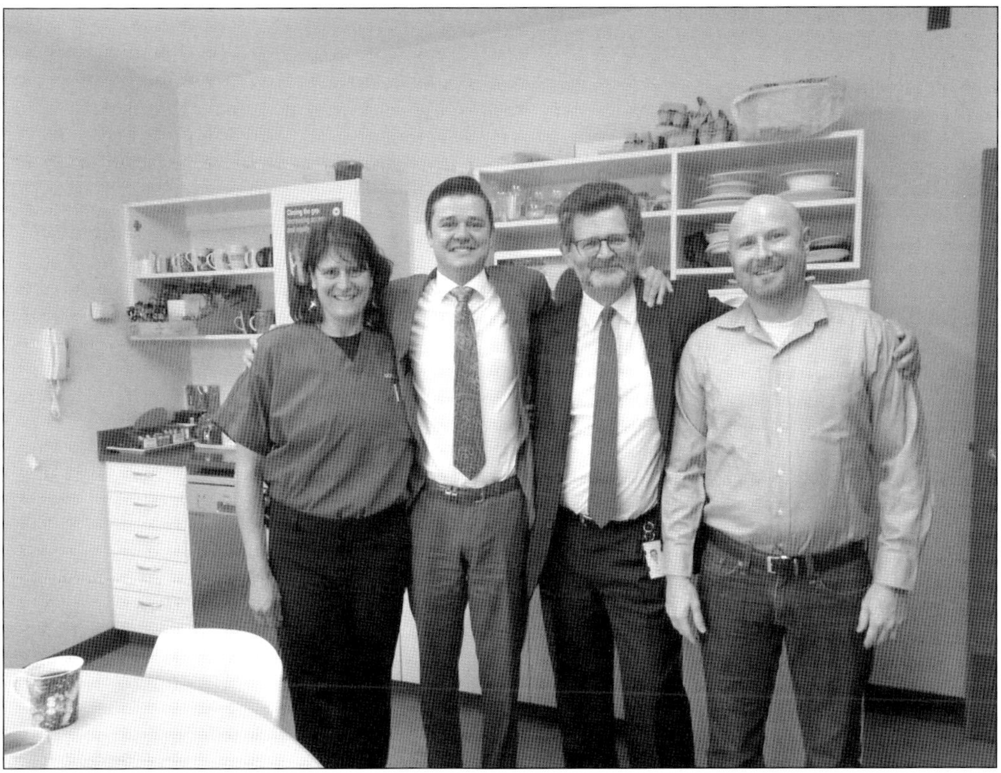

ER PAs in New Zealand. As the New Zealand pilot was completed, the employers of the "pilot PAs" hired other PAs to come to New Zealand and fill their slots. Lis Gammelin (left) worked as an emergency room PA in the small community of Gore on the South Island. MEDEX graduate Adam Wyble (Yakima 10, far right) took Gammelin's place when she returned to the United States in late 2014. Second and third from left are Karl Metzler, the leader of Gore-Health, and Tony Crane, the leader of the PA pilot for the Ministry of Health. (Author's collection.)

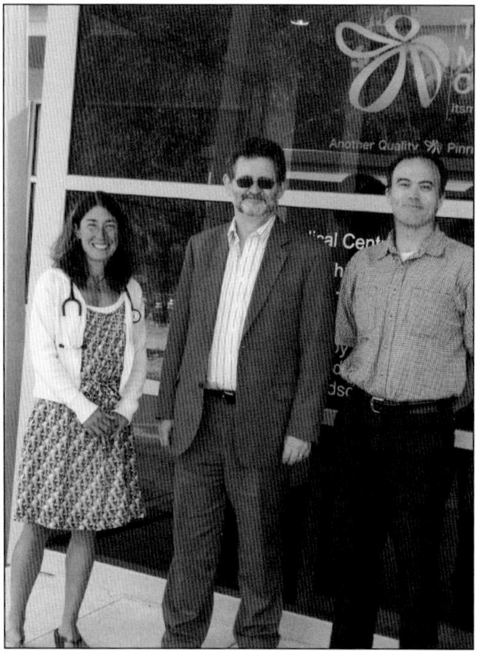

New Clinic in New Zealand. MEDEX graduates Amee Koch (Yakima 7, left) and Jeremy Palmer (Class 41, right) worked for Midlands Health in a newly built Tokorua clinic, which consolidated five general practices in Tokorua. Koch and Palmer are pictured at the entrance to the clinic with Tony Crane (center) from the Ministry of Health. (Author's collection.)

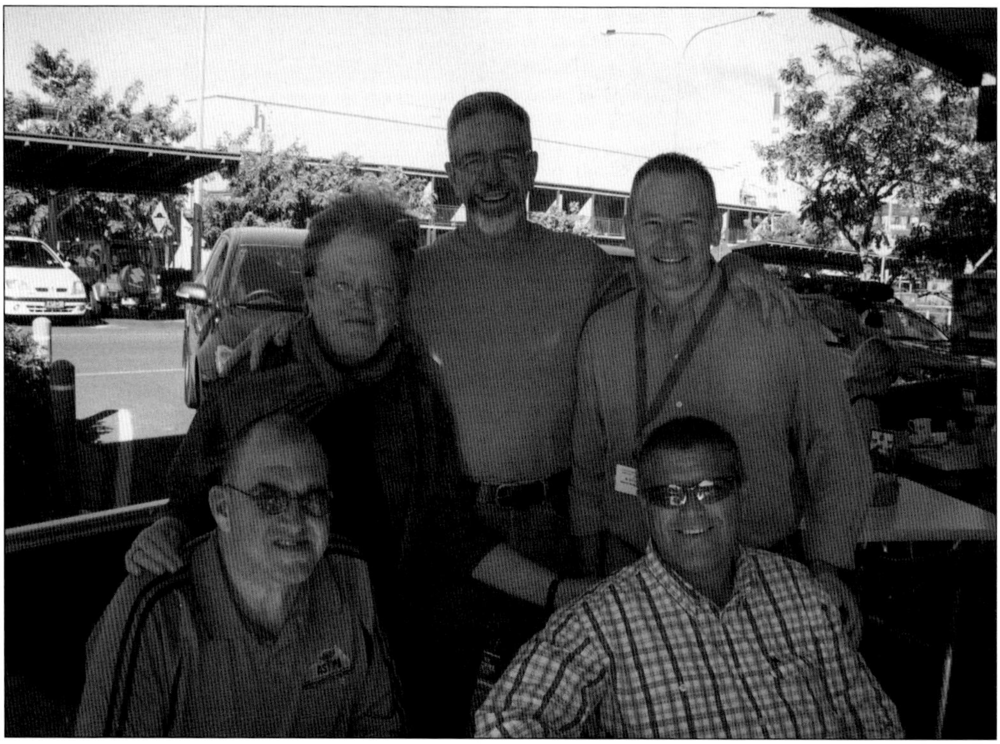

First Australian PA Students. Students in the first PA class at the University of Queensland are shown at a meeting of the Australian PA organization held in conjunction with the rural health conference, "Are You Remotely Interested?" in Mount Isa, Queensland. The photograph includes Al Forde in the center, director for the PA program at James Cook University, Townsville, and MEDEX director Ruth Ballweg, second from left. (Author's collection.)

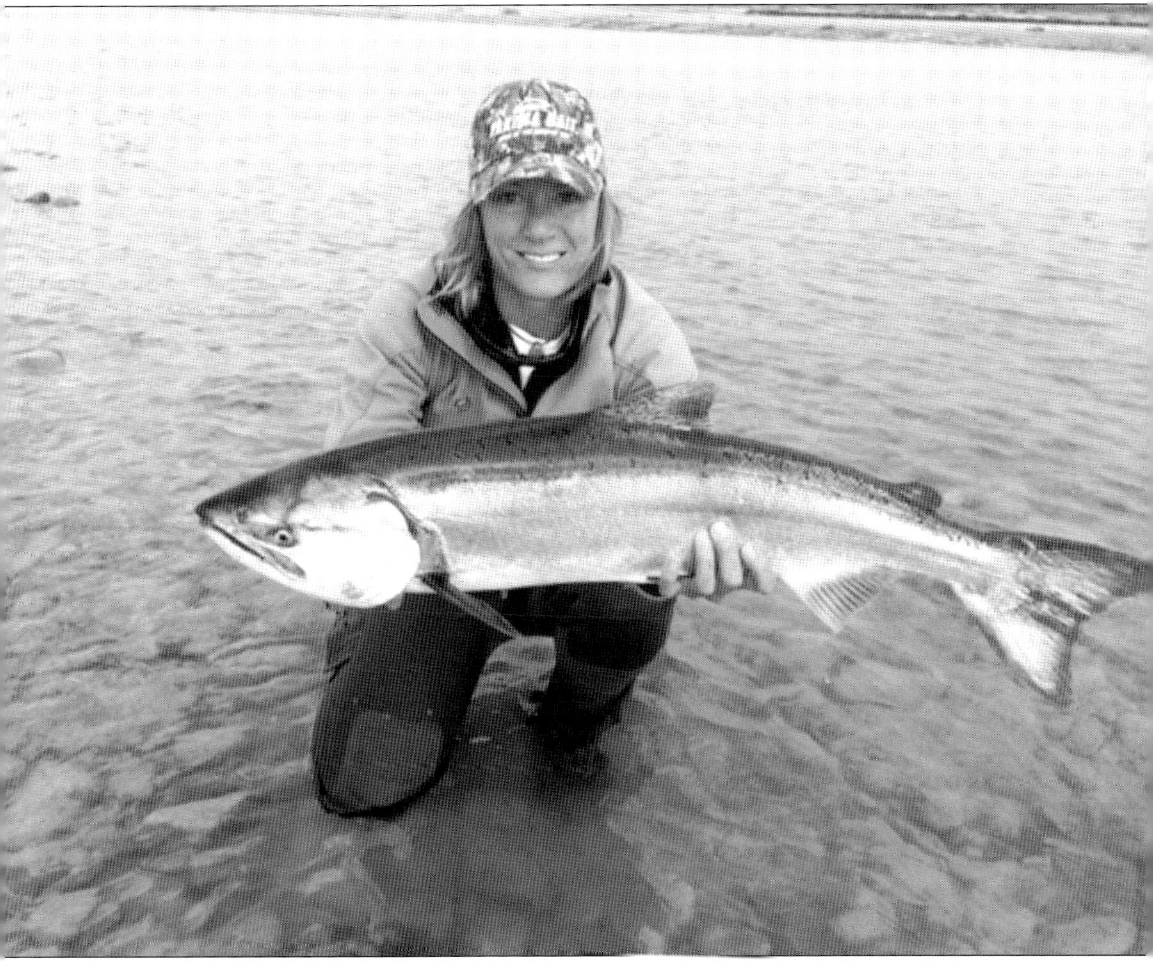

ENJOYING NEW ZEALAND. Machelle Dotson (Spokane 10) is pictured with her catch. (Courtesy of Machelle Dotson.)

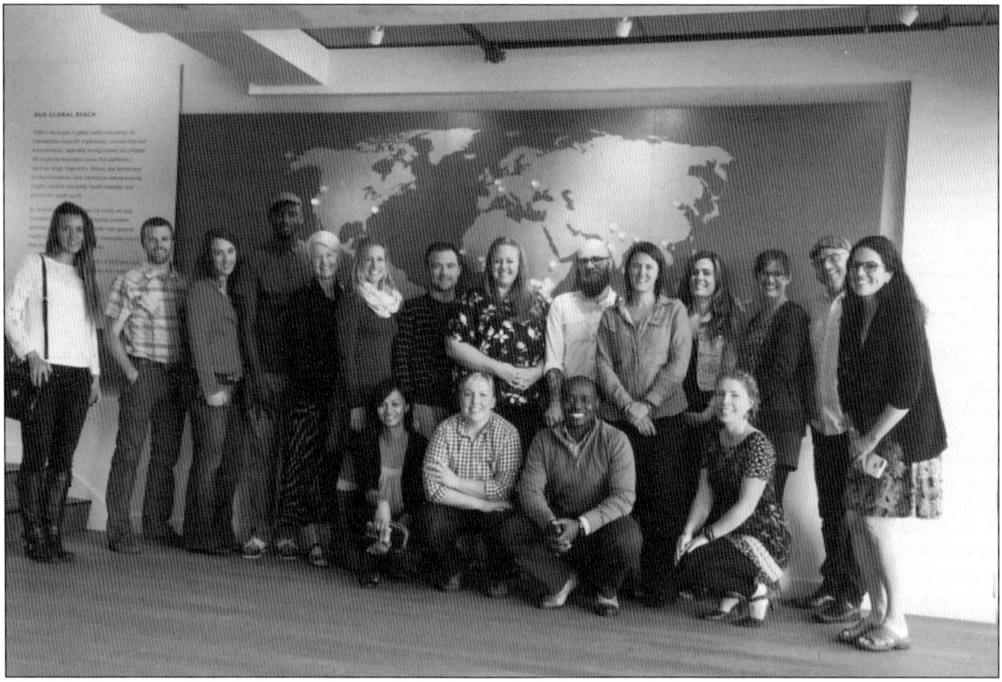

Global Health Pathway. The MEDEX master's degree in clinical health services includes the following four possible pathways: public health/prevention, academic medicine/specialty practice, primary care in rural and urban settings, and global health. MEDEX global students are pictured with course leaders and MEDEX faculty members Susan "Reba" McIntyre (fifth from left) and Alicia Quella (far right). (Courtesy of Susan McIntyre.)

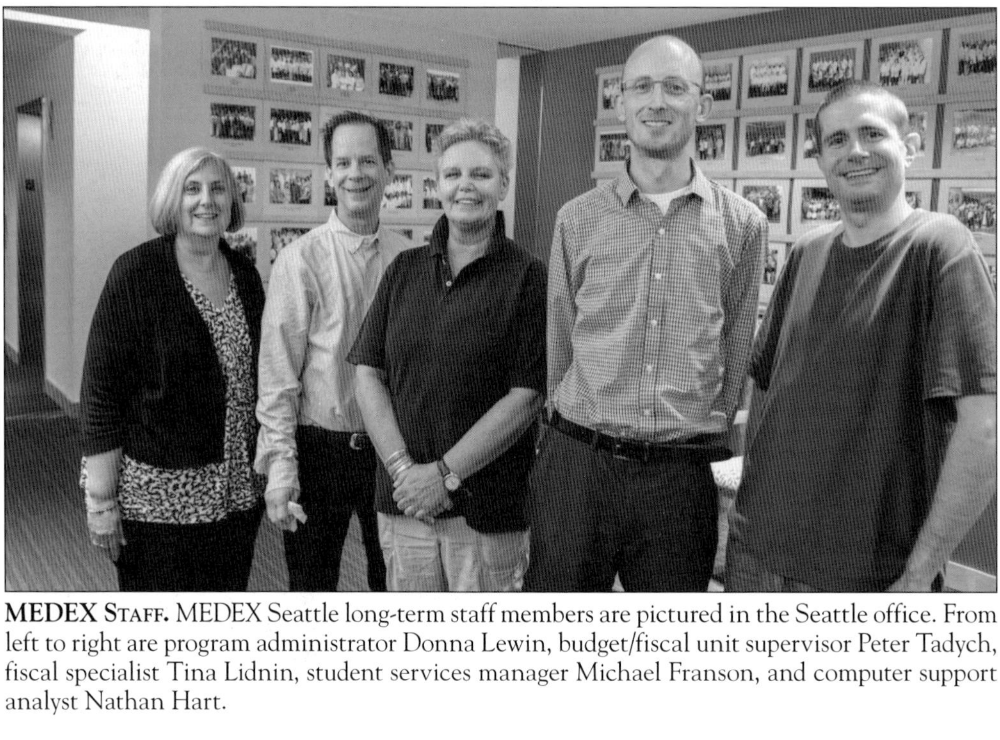

MEDEX Staff. MEDEX Seattle long-term staff members are pictured in the Seattle office. From left to right are program administrator Donna Lewin, budget/fiscal unit supervisor Peter Tadych, fiscal specialist Tina Lidnin, student services manager Michael Franson, and computer support analyst Nathan Hart.

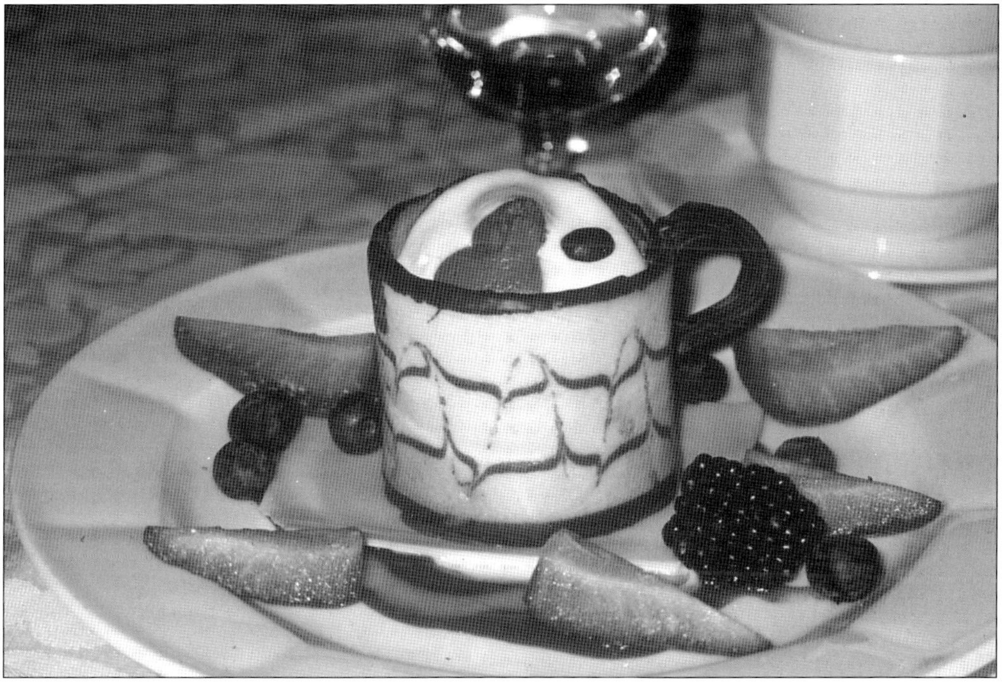

Have Hobby, Will Travel. Dr. Smith believes that effective advocates and clinicians should have a hobby. On his global travels, he favored the international language of chocolate, especially chocolate mousse. (This dessert, photographed by Ruth Ballweg, accompanied a meeting with Utah health-care providers.) A self-proclaimed tasting expert, Dr. Smith enjoys an extensive collection of pictures, recipes, and menus of memorable mousse-terpieces. (Author's collection.)

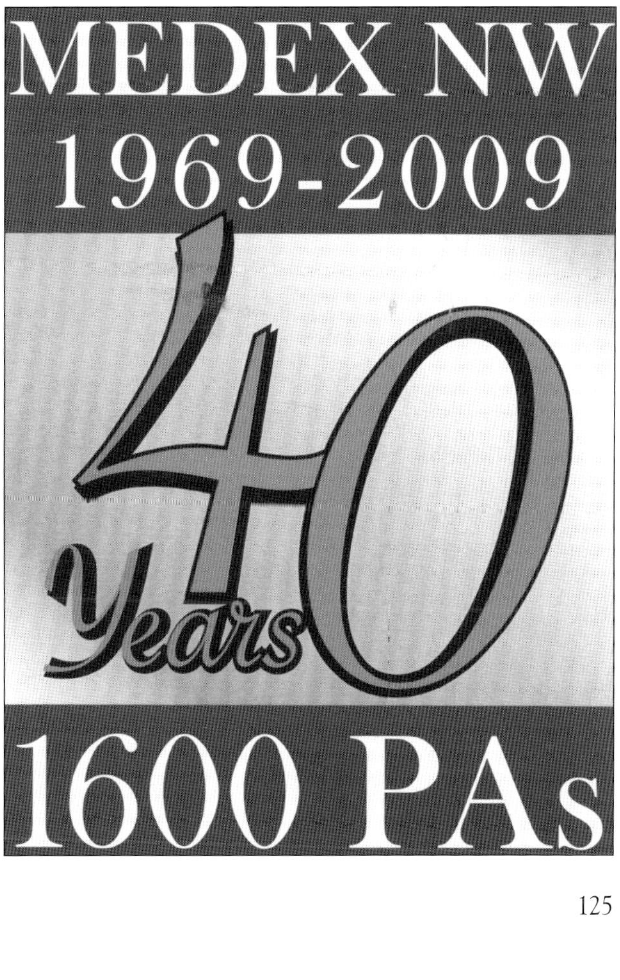

MEDEX Poster. This banner was designed for the MEDEX 40th anniversary celebration in 2009.

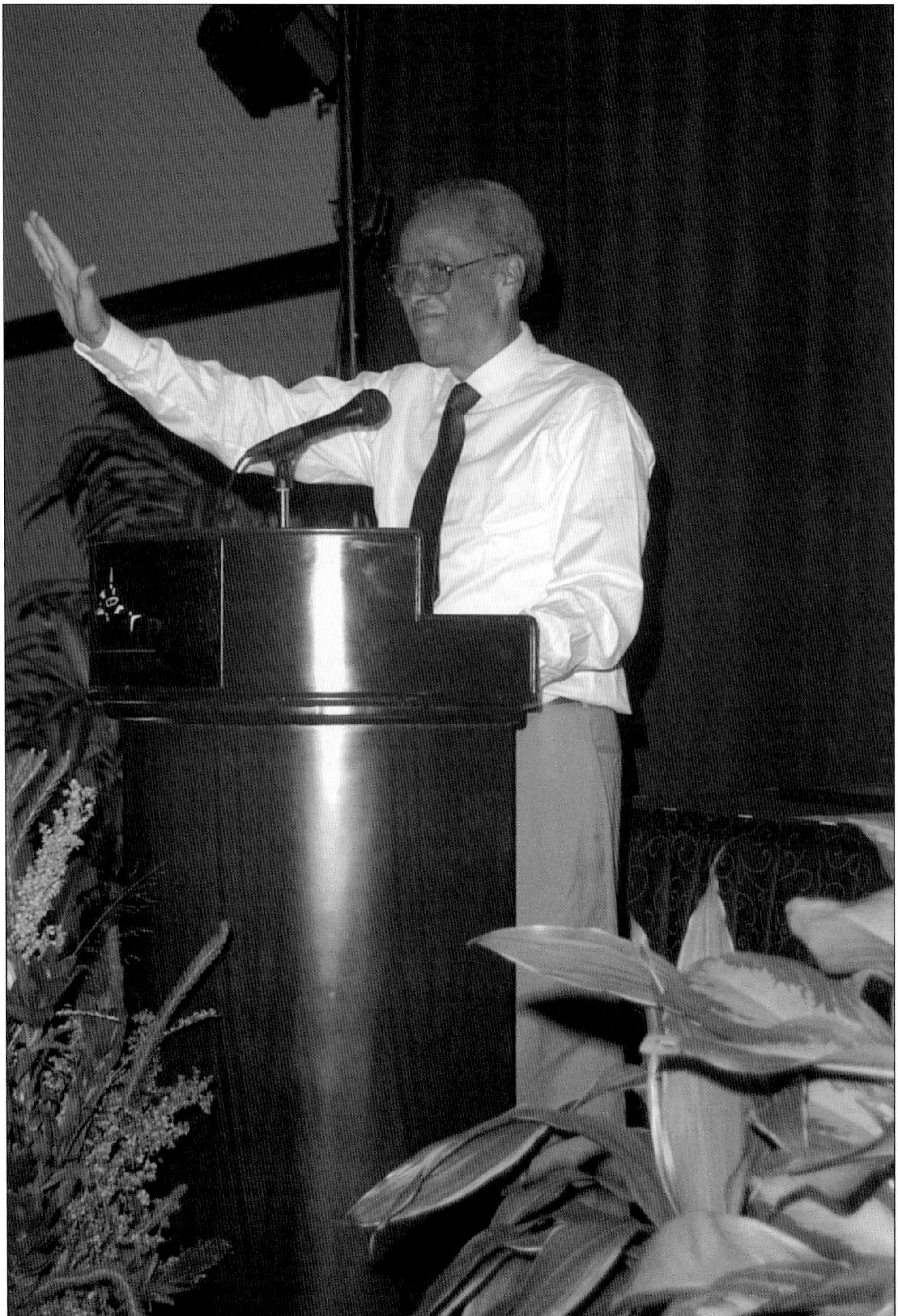

Celebration. MEDEX founder Dr. Richard Smith is pictured making final remarks at the MEDEX 40th anniversary celebration in 2009.

Bibliography

Ballweg, Ruth, Sherry Stolberg, and Edward Sullivan. *Physician Assistant: A Guide to Clinical Practice*. 1st ed. Philadelphia, PA: W.B. Saunders, 1994.

Ballweg, Ruth, Edward Sullivan, Darwin Brown, and Daniel Vetrosky. *Physician Assistant: A Guide to Clinical Practice*. 5th ed. Philadelphia, PA: W.B. Saunders, 2013.

Bliss, Ann, and Eva Cohen. *The New Health Professionals: Nurse Practitioners and Physician's Assistants*. Germantown, MD: Aspen Systems Corporation, 1976.

Bureau of Health Professions. *Physician Assistants in the Health Workforce 1994 Final Report of the Advisory Group on Physician Assistants and the Workforce*. Rockville, MD: US Department of Health and Human Services, 1994.

Carter, Reginald D., and Henry W. Perry. *Alternatives in Health Care Delivery: Emerging Roles for Physician Assistants*. St. Louis, MO: Warren Green Inc., 1984.

Clawson, D. Kay, and M. Osterweis. *The Roles of Physician Assistants and Nurse Practitioners in Primary Care*. Washington, DC: Association of Academic Health Centers, 1993.

Danielson, Randy, Ruth Ballweg, Linda Vorvick, and Donald Sefcik. *The Preceptors Guide to Supervising Physician Assistants*. Burlington, MA: Jones & Bartlett Learning, 2011.

Hooker, Roderick S., and James F. Cawley. *Physician Assistants in American Medicine*. New York, NY: Churchill Livingstone, 1997.

Myers, Hu C. *The Physician's Assistant: A Baccalaureate Curriculum*. Parsons, WV: McLain Printing Co., 1977.

Piemme, Thomas E., Alfred M. Sadler Jr., Reginald D. Carter, and Ruth Ballweg. *The Physician Assistant: An Illustrated History*. Atlanta, GA: Physician Assistant History Society, 2013.

Sadler, Alfred M. Jr., Blair L. Sadler, and Ann A. Bliss. *The Physician's Assistant Today and Tomorrow*. New Haven, CT: Yale University Press, 1972.

Schafft, Gretchen, and James F. Cawley. *The Physician Assistant in a Changing Health Care Environment*. Rockville, MD: Aspen Publishers, 1987.

Smith, Richard A. "MEDEX." *Journal of the American Medical Association*, March 16, 1970. 211 (11): 1842–1845.

———. "MEDEX: Five Years Later." *Journal of the American Medical Association*, July 14, 1975. 233 (2): 135–136.

Zarbock, Sarah, and Kenneth Harbert. *Physician Assistants: Present and Future Models of Utilization*. New York, NY: Praeger Publishers, 1986.